新医科英语系列教材

A COURSEBOOK OF ENGLISH FOR
MEDICAL HUMANITIES

医学人文英语教程

总主编◎黄立鹤　吴　赟

主　编◎李　芳

副主编◎田冬梅

编　者◎罗正鹏　黄　芳

　　　　赵忻怡　韩明月

清华大学出版社

北　京

内 容 简 介

本教材共 12 个单元，涵盖了医学人文领域中的核心学科和主题，包括医学史，医学哲学，医学伦理学，医学社会学，医学人类学，医学教育，叙事医学，文学、艺术与医学，新媒体与医学，医患交流，缓和医疗，以及健康素养等。每单元由三个部分构成，分别是学术广角、主题阅读和拓展阅读。每部分都包含一篇阅读文章和课后习题。通过阅读，学生可以了解各领域的基本概况、经典主题和学术前沿。习题设计包含语言、思维、学术层面的训练与考察，内容新颖，题型多样，有助于训练和提升学生的自主语言探索与批判性思维能力。

本教材适用于我国本科院校英语专业和公共英语教育教学，可以作为医学英语、学术英语或医学人文等相关课程教材使用，也可作为医学院校研究生公共英语教育教学资料使用。本教材配有优质音频资源，学生可直接扫码听音。

图书在版编目（CIP）数据

医学人文英语教程 / 黄立鹤，吴赟总主编；李芳主编 . —北京：清华大学出版社，2024.1
新医科英语系列教材
ISBN 978-7-302-64877-2

Ⅰ.①医…　Ⅱ.①黄…②吴…③李…　Ⅲ.①医学—人文科学—英语—教材　Ⅳ.①R

中国国家版本馆 CIP 数据核字（2023）第 215135 号

责任编辑：白周兵
封面设计：张伯阳
责任校对：王凤芝
责任印制：杨　艳

出版发行：清华大学出版社
　　　　　网　　　址：https://www.tup.com.cn, https://www.wqxuetang.com
　　　　　地　　　址：北京清华大学学研大厦 A 座　　　　邮　　编：100084
　　　　　社 总 机：010-83470000　　　　邮　　购：010-62786544
　　　　　投稿与读者服务：010-62776969，c-service@tup.tsinghua.edu.cn
　　　　　质量反馈：010-62772015，zhiliang@tup.tsinghua.edu.cn
印 装 者：三河市铭诚印务有限公司
经　　销：全国新华书店
开　　本：185mm×260mm　　　　**印　　张：**18.75　　　　**字　　数：**384 千字
版　　次：2024 年 1 月第 1 版　　　　**印　　次：**2024 年 1 月第 1 次印刷
定　　价：79.00 元

产品编号：099029-01

总　序

中华人民共和国成立以来，特别是改革开放以来，我国健康领域的改革发展取得了显著成就；近10年来，健康中国战略全面实施，人民健康得到全方位保障，我国走出了一条中国特色卫生健康事业改革发展之路。医学教育是卫生健康事业发展的重要基石，党的十八大以来，我国把人民健康放在优先发展的战略地位，医学教育蓬勃发展，高素质医学人才脱颖而出。面对实施健康中国战略的新任务、世界医学发展的新要求，我国仍需把医学教育摆在教育和卫生健康事业优先发展的地位。

随着我国持续推进卫生健康国际交流合作、深入参与全球卫生治理，健康医疗领域人员跨国界、跨地区流动已是大势所趋，国际化能力培养在我国医学教育发展中愈加受到重视。《国务院办公厅关于加快医学教育创新发展的指导意见》（国办发〔2020〕34号）（以下简称《指导意见》）明确指出，要"培养具有国际视野的高层次拔尖创新医学人才"。2020年6月，教育部临床医学专业认证工作委员会以"无条件通过"的结果正式获得世界医学教育联合会（World Federation of Medical Education，WFME）医学教育认证机构的认定，标志着我国医学教育标准和认证体系实现国际实质等效，医学教育认证质量得到了国际认可。毫无疑问，提升健康医学领域人才的国际化视野和能力是落实我国"新医科"教育理念的重要方面。

为进一步落实"新医科"教育中的国际化能力培养，提升健康医学专业学生的英语应用能力，我们深度参与了"新医科英语系列教材"的编撰工作，主要承担《医学英语基础教程》《医学英语阅读教程》《医学英语写作教程》《医学人文英语教程》《临床医学英语教程》《中医药英语实用教程》等教材的编写。本套教材围绕与健康医学相关的众多议题，落实加快以疾病治疗为中心向以健康促进为中心的转变，体现"大健康"理念，覆盖基础医学、临床医学、中医药、医学技术、公共卫生、医学人文、医学史、医学哲学等各类题材，涉及健康医学领域的核心范畴、前沿技术、行业标准、历史文化、健康治理等内容。体裁丰富多样，包含说明文、议论文、记叙文、应用文及人物访谈等。教材构思新颖，如把语块教学理念融入基础语言教学，设置真实医学临床实践和研究场景的英语教学，凸显基于医学英语任务的思辨创新能力培养，启发不同健康医学活动背后的跨文化思考，引导学生利用网络信息平台查找专业信息，介绍医工、医理、医文等学科交叉融合的前沿内容等。练习形式有趣、内涵丰富，要求学生对健康医学领域的实际问题进行创新性解决，从而实现英语语言能力和医药卫生专业视野的双向拓展。

全面推进课程思政建设是落实立德树人根本任务的战略举措。《指导意见》明确指出，要"强化医学生职业素养教育，加强医学伦理、科研诚信教育，发挥课程思政作用"，从而培养仁心仁术的医学人才。在编写中，我们始终牢记英语教学的育人功能，融入中国立场、价值伦理、职业素养等内容，潜移默化地引导学生逐步树立良好医德。我们努力平衡语言难度、学术深度、人文温度、历史厚度，在医学科学与语言人文中寻找结合点，力图打造一套既能体现医学人文思想，又兼具国际视野和家国情怀的高水平医学英语教材。

本套教材参照教育部《大学英语教学指南（2020版）》的课程设置要求，兼顾专门用途英语和通用英语；同时，参考《高等职业教育专科英语课程标准（2021年版）》，兼顾英语课程结构中的基础模块和拓展模块。因此，本套教材呈现一定的难度进阶，既可以作为应用型本科或高职高专医药卫生类专业的英语教材，也可作为普通高校本科阶段大学英语教学中的医学专门用途英语教材，个别教材甚至可用于英语类专业课堂教学或课后阅读材料使用；同时，它在一定程度上还适合愿意学习国际健康医学相关内容的社会人士，可满足临床医学、护理、药学、医学技术、卫生管理等方向的英语学习需要。

本套教材由同济大学发起，联合北京大学、山东大学、陕西师范大学、扬州大学、黑龙江大学、曲阜师范大学、四川外国语大学、上海中医药大学（及附属龙华医院）、天津中医药大学、广西医科大学、济宁医学院、南京工业职业技术大学、山东医学高等专科学校等高校，邀请医学英语教学、健康话语研究等领域内经验丰富的专家、教师和医生充分研讨、共同编写而成。同济以医学建校，学校始于1907年德国医生埃里希·宝隆在中德两国政府和社会各界支持下创办的医学堂，走的是一条由医而工，再到综合的发展之路。学校虽于20世纪50年代在全国高校院系布局调整中将医学院整体迁至武汉，但同济人医学情结至深，历经百年沧桑后，在新世纪之初重建医学。近年来，同济医科勇闯创新发展之路，结合世界医学发展前沿、未来趋势及国家需求，加快向国际一流水准迈进。

我们衷心希望本套教材能够配合深化医学教育改革，协助推进"卓越医生教育培养计划 2.0"，帮助学习者实现英语语言能力与医药卫生专业视野的双向拓展，培养其在健康医学领域进行国际交流合作的能力，使其成为我国推进卫生健康国际交流合作、参与全球卫生治理的重要人才。

黄立鹤　吴赟

2023 年 6 月于上海同济园

前　言

党的二十大报告指出，为了全面推进中华民族伟大复兴，我们要"实施科教兴国战略，强化现代化建设人才支撑"。"教育是国之大计、党之大计"，加强教材建设和管理是完善高质量教育体系改革的重要环节。在二十大精神的指引下，本教材在深刻领会和贯穿课程思政理念的基础上，以博览世界科学精华、弘扬社会主义核心价值观为基本目标，选取了兼具"科学性、前沿性、人文性"的文本素材，设计了具有"探索、反思、实践"特色的习题，引导学生挖掘具有中华民族特色的医药健康文化与经验，启发学生用英语来讲述中国医药与健康文化故事，树立其民族文化自信以及为建设人类健康命运共同体而奋斗的理想与信念。

依据"新医科""新文科"指导思想，本教材以医学人文学科基础为依托，选取世界范围内医学人文经典主题和前沿话题相关英语文献材料，通过引导式阅读、启发式反思和创新性思维等相关阅读活动设计，带领学生了解医学人文基本内涵、饱览医学人文学科成果、学习与反思医学人文在临床实践中的意义。本教材共涵盖 12 个主题单元，每单元由三个部分构成，每部分都包含一篇阅读文章和相关习题。其中，第一部分是"学术广角"（Academic Horizon），该部分选用的文章主要是介绍相关学术领域的定义、内容和范畴，为学生提供一个学术概况与背景介绍；习题以启发思考为主。第二部分是"主题阅读"（Thematic Reading），也是每单元的核心学习内容。该部分通常是围绕本领域内重要的、具有里程碑意义的人物、事件或历史时刻等展开的阅读材料，旨在启迪和引导学生对本领域相关问题进行深入思考与探索；习题设计丰富，覆盖语言、文化、思维等多层次的训练。第三部分是"拓展阅读"（Extended Reading），所选文章也是相关领域内具有代表性的阅读材料，文本兼具实用性和思考性；习题以口语表达和反思性写作训练为主。

本教材具有以下特色：

一、展示医学人文前沿成果，突出学术性特色

本教材编者大多具有丰富的医学人文教研经验，编写内容丰富、全面，具有代表性。本教材涵盖了医学史、医学哲学、医学伦理学、医学社会学、医学人类学、叙事医学等医学人文领域核心主流学科的学术概况与经典文本，可以使学生实现"一卷在手，胜读百卷"的愿望。除了在内容上具有人文属性之外，本教材的设计也凸显了人文特征。每单元都由一句能体现该领域特色的经典名言引入，并配有一幅世界医学与人文领域著名油画作品，使学生在阅读文本之前就与该领域产生直观、生动、形象的联结，带有敬畏之情和真诚之意去开启阅读的征程。每单元课后习题的设计以开放性题目为主，为学生的自我探索和发挥提供空间。此外，本教材还打破以往阅读命题的传统，设计了包含辩论、演讲、角色扮演等在内的多样化语言与思维训练习题，以及"小型研究项目"等学术启蒙专项练习，引导学生通过研究深入了解医学人文领域，逐步开启学术发展之路。因此，本教材可谓是一把打开通往医学人文学术大门的钥匙。

二、秉承以内容为依托、以产出为导向的教育理念，强调自主性特色

近年来，为了适应新时代英语教学改革的需求，"以内容为依托、以产出为导向"的语言教育理念越来越得到广泛的认可和应用。本教材通过选用医学人文领域的基础和经典文本为阅读材料，实现了"以内容为依托"的教材设计，使学生在了解和阅读医学人文内容的过程中输入英语语言元素；并通过设计多层次、多样化的课后习题，从语言积累到思考讨论，再到口头和书面表达等多方位实现"以产出为导向"的语言输出目标。为了培养学生的自主语言学习能力，本教材在习题中融入渐进引导式设计理念。语言类训练以开放性题目为主，习题设计纵向体现了词汇、词组、语句的习得顺序，横向引入从泛学到精学、从输入到输出的学习理念。在泛学词汇练习中要求学生建立自己的"泛学词汇表"，并引导学生对所选词汇进行归类整理；在精学词汇模块，学生可以在学习中英文释义后根据自身情况对每个单词进行评价，充分调动学生在单词学习环节的自主性。在选词填空题目中，本教材前六个单元同时提供英文语句和中文翻译，后六个单元仅保留英文语句，便于学生逐步锻炼和提升语境辨析能力。因此，本教材可谓是面向学生开放的一段自主语言学习与探索之旅。

三、提升批判性、创新性思维能力，彰显开放性特色

语言与思维之间的关系密不可分，思维能力培养是外语教学中不可或缺的环节。为了支持我国创新型人才培养目标，提升学生的批判性、创新性思维能力，本教材坚持贯穿阅读、探索、反思三位一体的思想，通过多层次、多维度、多界面的阅读活动设计引导学生结合所读内容主动展开研习和探索，并帮助他们基于探索结果进行反思和总结。例如，在阅读"医师职业精神"相关内容后，本教材启发学生对"中国人眼中的理想医生"进行调研，以研究报告的形式整理调研结果，并对标国际医师职业精神标准进行反思性书写；再如，在阅读"文化与健康"相关内容后，本教材安排学生进行角色扮演，表演中医大夫与外国病人之间看病就医的场景，反思中医特色与精华，学习如何用英语传递中医文化精髓。我们希望，本教材能够为学生打开一扇体现医学人文思想、兼具国际视野和家国情怀的全新思考之窗。

本教材的读者对象包括医药卫生类专业学生，以及有意愿学习医学人文相关内容、渴望提升学术英语水平的其他学习者。通过本教材的学习，学生不仅会提高英语语言阅读理解能力和批判性、创新性思维能力，而且还将全面提升自身的医学人文素养，为后期在医学领域的职业发展奠定深厚的人文基础。尽管编者已尽心，但百密一疏，难免还有不周之处，我们诚邀广大读者多提建议、不吝赐教，以期不断完善。

李芳　田冬梅

2023 年 12 月于北京

Contents

Unit 1 History of Medicine

> We are not makers of history. We are made by history.
> —Martin Luther King Jr.

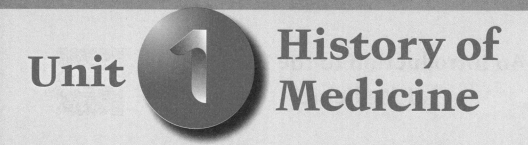

The Agnew Clinic, by Thomas Eakins, 1889

Part 1 Academic Horizon

An Introduction to the History of Medicine[①]

Medicine touches us all at some stage in our lives. Whether we live in a crowded high-tech industrialized society that uses the diagnostic and **therapeutic** tools of modern bioscience or in an isolated rural community where health care is perhaps less formal, less **intrusive** and less commercial, it is arguably medicine, rather than religion or law, that **dictates** the manner in which we are born, the quality of our lives, and the ease and speed of our deaths. Indeed, although modern populations are increasingly struggling to **cope with chronic** conditions, such as cancer, heart disease, **arthritis**, obesity and depression, we have come to rely heavily on the ability of medicine to help us live relatively happily, healthily and productively well into our eighties.

Given the extent to which it **penetrates** the physical, psychological and even spiritual **dimensions** of human existence, it is no surprise that medicine constitutes a vast **territory**. In the early 21st century, the practice of medicine **incorporates**, among other things, the **preservation** of health and the prevention of illness, the discovery and application of **pharmacological** tools to **combat** mental and physical disease,

New Expressions	
therapeutic /ˌθerə'pjuːtɪk/ *adj.* 治疗的；医疗的；治病的	**penetrate** /'penətreɪt/ *v.* 渗透，打入（组织、团体等）
intrusive /ɪn'truːsɪv/ *adj.* 侵入的；闯入的；侵扰的；烦扰的	**dimension** /daɪ'menʃn/ *n.* 方面；侧面；维度
dictate /'dɪkteɪt/ *v.* 支配；摆布；决定	**territory** /'terətɔːri/ *n.* 领土；版图；领地
cope with 处理；应付	**incorporate** /ɪn'kɔːrpəreɪt/ *v.* 将……包括在内；包含；吸收；使并入
chronic /'krɑːnɪk/ *adj.* 长期的；慢性的；难以治愈（或根除）的	**preservation** /ˌprezər'veɪʃn/ *n.* 保护；维护；保存
arthritis /ɑːr'θraɪtɪs/ *n.* 关节炎	**pharmacological** /ˌfɑːrməkə'lɑːdʒɪkl/ *adj.* 药理学的
	combat /'kɑːmbæt/ *v.* 防止；减轻

---

① The text is adapted from the following source: Jackson, M. 2014. *The History of Medicine: A Beginner's Guide.* New York: Simon and Schuster.

 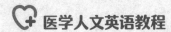

the development of novel diagnostic and **surgical** techniques to identify and remove **tumors**, heal broken bones or restore blood-flow to **ailing** hearts, the **formulation** of policies designed to protect national and global public health, the use of **psychotherapy**[1] to reduce depression and anxiety and to **promote** happiness, the **delivery** of welfare services and medical support to mothers and their children, and the **alleviation** of pain and **disability**.

In the past, the **contours** of medicine have been even more **expansive**. In both Eastern and Western cultures, medicine has embraced religion, magic, **alchemy** and **astrology**, as well as the application of **herbal remedies**, the use of **healing rituals**, sacrifices and offerings to the gods, and the relief of poverty. Health care has been dispensed not only in **specialist** institutions, including hospitals, **workhouses**, **monasteries** and **hospices**, but also regularly in the community, on the battlefield and at home. Within these diverse environments, advice and **treatment** were delivered by a range of practitioners often trained in quite different ways and **possessing** different, although usually **complementary**, skills and knowledge. In sickness and in health, patients sought the services of **shamans**, **diviners**, **priests**, **midwives**, nurses, **physicians**,

New Expressions	
surgical /'sɜːrdʒɪkl/ *adj.* 外科的；外科手术的	**specialist** /'speʃəlɪst/ *n.* 专家；专科医生
tumor /'tuːmər/ *n.* 瘤；肿瘤；肿块	**workhouse** /'wɜːrkhaʊs/ *n.*（英国旧时的）济贫院，劳动救济所
ailing /'eɪlɪŋ/ *adj.* 有病的；体弱的	
formulation /ˌfɔːrmjuˈleɪʃn/ *n.*（政策、计划等的）制定，制订	**monastery** /'mɑːnəsteri/ *n.* 隐修院；修道院；寺院
promote /prəˈmoʊt/ *v.* 促进；推动	**hospice** /'hɑːspɪs/ *n.* 临终安养院
delivery /dɪˈlɪvəri/ *n.* 传送；递送；交付	**treatment** /'triːtmənt/ *n.* 治疗；疗法；诊治；护理
alleviation /əˌliːviˈeɪʃn/ *n.* 减轻；缓和；缓解	
disability /ˌdɪsəˈbɪləti/ *n.*（指状态、身心、学习等方面的）缺陷，障碍	**possess** /pəˈzes/ *v.* 有；拥有
contour /'kɑːntʊr/ *n.* 外形；轮廓	**complementary** /ˌkɑːmplɪˈmentri/ *adj.* 互补的；补充的；相互补足的
expansive /ɪkˈspænsɪv/ *adj.* 广泛的；全面的	**shaman** /'ʃɑːmən/ *n.* 萨满（据信能和善恶神灵沟通、能治病的人）
alchemy /'ælkəmi/ *n.* 炼金术	
astrology /əˈstrɑːlədʒi/ *n.* 占星术；占星学	**diviner** /dɪˈvaɪnə/ *n.* 预言者；占卜者；推测者
herbal /'hɜːrbl/ *adj.* 药草的	**priest** /priːst/ *n.*（天主教、圣公会、东正教的）司祭，神父，司铎
remedy /'remədi/ *n.* 疗法；治疗，药品	
healing /'hiːlɪŋ/ *n.* 康复	**midwife** /'mɪdwaɪf/ *n.* 助产士；接生员；产婆
ritual /'rɪtʃuəl/ *n.* 程序；仪规；礼节；（尤指）宗教仪式	**physician** /fɪˈzɪʃn/ *n.* 医师；（尤指）内科医生

surgeons, **apothecaries**, and a **miscellany** of **itinerant** practitioners, **charlatans** and **quacks**. Historically, medicine has never constituted a **monolithic** system of knowledge and practice but has always been marked by a **vibrant** sense of diversity and **pluralism**. The task of **unraveling** the history of medicine is further complicated by the fact that medical theory and practice, as well as the **distribution** and patterns of disease, have been so deeply **embedded** in social contexts that the boundary between medicine and society has been **indiscernible**. In all ages and all cultures, the appearance, spread and control of both infectious and non-infectious diseases have been dictated by social, economic and cultural factors. At the same time, the practice of medicine has been a social **endeavor**, not only reflecting the norms and expectations of patients and politicians alike but also influencing the beliefs, **customs** and hopes of the sick, the healthy and their healers. Even in the modern era of **biomedicine**[2], when science appears to offer a more objective perspective on health and illness, scientific knowledge, clinical practice and health care policies continue to be determined by social and cultural factors as well as economic and political **expediency**.

There has been a tendency in recent times to **distinguish** rather deliberately between science and the humanities, as if they possess entirely different agendas and methods or **constitute** entirely different intellectual cultures. While science and medicine appear to offer more reliable **accounts** of the natural world and its problems, the

New Expressions

apothecary /ə'pɑːθəkeri/ *n.*（旧时制药兼售药的）药剂师，药商

miscellany /'mɪsəleɪni/ *n.* 杂集；混合体

itinerant /aɪ'tɪnərənt/ *adj.* 巡回的；流动的；（尤指为找工作）四处奔波的

charlatan /'ʃɑːrlətən/ *n.* 假充内行的人；骗子

quack /kwæk/ *n.* 江湖郎中；冒牌医生；庸医

monolithic /ˌmɑːnə'lɪθɪk/ *adj.* 整体的

vibrant /'vaɪbrənt/ *adj.* 充满生机的；生机勃勃的；精力充沛的

pluralism /'plʊrəlɪzəm/ *n.* 多元化，多元性（不同种族、不同政治或宗教信仰的多种群体共存）

unravel /ʌn'rævl/ *v.* 阐释；说明；澄清；变得清楚易懂

distribution /ˌdɪstrɪ'bjuːʃn/ *n.* 分配；分布

embedded /ɪm'bedɪd/ *adj.* 被牢牢地嵌入（或插入、埋入）……中

indiscernible /ˌɪndɪ'sɜːrnəbl/ *adj.* 隐约的；依稀的；不明显的

endeavor /ɪn'devər/ *n.*（尤指新的或艰苦的）努力，尝试

custom /'kʌstəm/ *n.*（个人的）习惯，习性，惯常行为

expediency /ɪk'spiːdiənsi/ *n.* 权宜之计

distinguish /dɪ'stɪŋɡwɪʃ/ *v.* 区分；辨别；分清

constitute /'kɑːnstətuːt/ *v.* 组成；构成

account /ə'kaʊnt/ *n.*（思想、理论、过程的）解释，说明，叙述

humanities seem to deal only with subjective, and often **unverifiable**, aspects of personal and public life. As a result, historical, philosophical or **literary** studies of medicine and science have often been **divorced** from the pursuit of clinical knowledge, improved health policies and better treatments. For a number of reasons, it is a mistake to impose a **distinction** between medicine and history in this way. In the first instance, the **notion** of history has always been **integral** to clinical methods. From ancient to modern medicine, students have been taught to consider the patient's history from various perspectives: the history of current symptoms; the patient's past medical, **occupational** and social history; and the family (and increasingly this means **genetic**) history. Personal and biological, as well as collective and **psychosocial**, histories have thus been central to the processes of accurately diagnosing disease and formulating appropriate treatments and policies. Second, as both historians and doctors have pointed out, history also constitutes a **vehicle** for educating, inspiring and humanizing medical and nursing students who might otherwise **succumb** to the **brutalizing** effects of regular **exposure** to disease and death.

Perhaps more **contentiously**, research in the **medical humanities**[3] allows us to recognize the power and limits of medicine and to **acknowledge** the cultural, social and political, rather than merely technical, obstacles to **health promotion**[4] and disease prevention. By exploring the human aspects of medicine and tracing the development of medical theories, policies and institutions across time, medical history can reveal the manner in which medicine reflects and shapes far wider historical currents and the extent to which experiences of health and disease structure our lives. More

New Expressions	
unverifiable /ˌʌnˌverəˈfaɪəbl/ adj. 无法核实的；无法检验的；不能证实的	**vehicle** /ˈviːəkl/ n.（赖以表达思想、感情或达到目的的）手段，工具
literary /ˈlɪtəreri/ adj. 文学的	**succumb** /səˈkʌm/ v. 屈服；屈从；抵挡不住（攻击、疾病、诱惑等）
divorce /dɪˈvɔːrs/ v. 使分离；使脱离	
distinction /dɪˈstɪŋkʃn/ n. 差别；区别；对比	**brutalize** /ˈbruːtəlaɪz/ v. 使丧失人类情感；使变残忍
notion /ˈnoʊʃn/ n. 观念；信念；理解	**exposure** /ɪkˈspoʊʒər/ n. 面临，遭受（危险或不快）
integral /ˈɪntɪɡrəl/ adj. 必需的；不可或缺的	
occupational /ˌɑːkjuˈpeɪʃənl/ adj. 职业的	**contentiously** /kənˈtenʃəsli/ adv. 可能引起争论地
genetic /dʒəˈnetɪk/ adj. 基因的；遗传学的	
psychosocial /ˌsaɪkouˈsouʃl/ adj. 社会心理的（指社会环境影响下的个人心理变化）	**acknowledge** /əkˈnɑːlɪdʒ/ v. 承认（属实）

broadly, while science can uncover many of the **mechanisms** underlying patterns of health and disease, it is the humanities that can more effectively reveal the meanings of our experiences of pain and suffering. Medical history and the wider humanities, like the **biomedical** sciences, should therefore be integral to our search for health and happiness.

Historians have approached the history of medicine in different ways. Some scholars have focused on **narrating** and celebrating great discoveries made by **pioneers** in the field or on the health and illnesses of key historical figures. In these stories of **progressive innovation**, the achievements of Hippocrates[5], Galen[6], Ibn Sina[7], Ambroise Paré[8], Andreas Vesalius[9], William Harvey[10], Edward Jenner[11], John Snow[12], Ignaz Semmelweis[13], Florence Nightingale[14], Joseph Lister[15], Louis Pasteur[16], Robert Koch[17], Alexander Fleming[18] and many others have taken center stage. Such tales of success are not without **merit**: They highlight the extraordinary contributions of doctors to the history of humankind and bring the drama and significance of medicine to the **fore**. At the same time, however, they often give **precedence** to the **accomplishments** of men over women, the traditions of the West over the East, and the importance of biological and technological, rather than social and cultural, factors.

By contrast, social historians have recently moved away from telling stories of **triumphal** progress towards an approach that emphasizes the historical **contingency** of medical knowledge and the cultural specificity of experiences of health and illness. In these histories, there is no **fundamental** or enduring truth waiting to be unearthed by **enlightened** scientists and doctors; rather, knowledge and practice are regarded as always

---

New Expressions

mechanism /ˈmekənɪzəm/ *n.* 方法；机制

biomedical /ˌbaɪoʊˈmedɪkl/ *adj.* 生物医学的

narrate /ˈnæreɪt/ *v.* 讲（故事）；叙述

pioneer /ˌpaɪəˈnɪr/ *n.* 先锋；先驱；带头人

progressive /prəˈgresɪv/ *adj.* 进步的；先进的

innovation /ˌɪnəˈveɪʃn/ *n.*（新事物、思想或方法的）创造；创新；改革

merit /ˈmerɪt/ *n.* 优点；美德；价值

fore /fɔːr/ *n.* 变得重要（或突出）；起重要作用

precedence /ˈpresɪdəns/ *n.* 优先；优先权

accomplishment /əˈkɑːmplɪʃmənt/ *n.* 成就；成绩

triumphal /traɪˈʌmfl/ *adj.* 庆祝成功（或胜利）的；凯旋的

contingency /kənˈtɪndʒənsi/ *n.* 可能发生的事；偶发（或不测、意外）事件

fundamental /ˌfʌndəˈmentl/ *adj.* 基础的；基本的

enlightened /ɪnˈlaɪtnd/ *adj.* 开明的；有见识的；摆脱偏见的

shifting, and contested, products of socio-cultural and political forces. While such accounts of medicine and disease in the past effectively reveal the social determinants of health and healing, they tend to lose the sense of theater and urgency embedded in the practice of medicine and to ignore the extent to which both past and present populations have routinely depended on medicine to forge a better world.

History not only reveals elements of continuity and change in medical theory and practice but also exposes the close relationship between personal experiences of illness, scientific knowledge of bodies and minds, and the broader social factors that influence our understandings of health and disease. In addition, historical research clearly demonstrates shifting attitudes to the complex interactions among patients, doctors and disease.

The changing successions of errors and victories constitute the very essence of our history, which leads us, by paths that are sometimes luminous and at other times barely discernible, to laws that today seem impregnable and yesterday seemed vague and distant; to doubts that yesterday were dogmas, to hypotheses that perhaps tomorrow will be truths. To study this process of evolution in medicine; to scrutinize the distant origins and structure of our knowledge, formed slowly and painfully through so many and such different paths; to recognize after strict analysis the part that was played in the formation of medical thought by instinct, fear, hope, and faith, and the influence on this thought of the great events of political and social history; to measure the effect of medicine, on its side, in determining the direction of the history of culture, art, politics, social life; to endeavor finally to tie the present logically and harmoniously to the past—this should be the program of the history of medicine.

New Expressions	
shifting /'ʃɪftɪŋ/ *adj.* 移动的；狡诈的	**discernible** /dɪ'sɜːrnəbl/ *adj.* 可识别的
contest /kən'test/ *v.* 争辩；提出异议	**impregnable** /ɪm'pregnəbl/ *adj.* 坚不可摧的；牢不可破的
determinant /dɪ'tɜːrmɪnənt/ *n.* 决定因素；决定条件	**vague** /veɪg/ *adj.* 不清楚的；模糊的；朦胧的
expose /ɪk'spoʊz/ *v.* 暴露；显露	**dogma** /'dɔːgmə/ *n.* 教义；教理；信条；教条
demonstrate /'demənstreɪt/ *v.* 证明；证实；论证；说明	**scrutinize** /'skruːtənaɪz/ *v.* 仔细查看；认真检查；细致审查
essence /'esns/ *n.* 本质；实质；精髓	**instinct** /'ɪnstɪŋkt/ *n.* 本能；天性
luminous /'luːmɪnəs/ *adj.* 夜光的；发光的；发亮的	**harmoniously** /hɑːr'moʊniəsli/ *adv.* 和谐地

1. **psychotherapy:** 心理治疗。心理治疗是心理学术语，指通过与精神科医生、心理学家或其他心理健康从业者交谈，以治疗心理健康问题。During psychotherapy, clients learn about their conditions, moods, feelings, thoughts and behaviors.

2. **biomedicine:** 生物医学。生物医学强调通过生物学研究验证的标准化、循证治疗方法，由经过正规培训的医生、护士和其他执业医师进行治疗。近一个世纪以来，生物医学一直是西方的主导医学体系。Biomedicine is a branch of medical science that applies biological and physiological principles to clinical practice.

3. **medical humanities:** 医学人文。医学人文学科使用跨学科研究来探索健康和疾病的体验，通常侧重于主观的或无形的体验。这种跨学科的属性使该领域具有多样性，并鼓励创造性的"认识论创新"。Medical humanity is an interdisciplinary field of medicine which includes the humanities (philosophy, ethics, history, comparative literature and religion), social sciences (psychology, sociology, anthropology, cultural studies and health geography) and the arts (literature, theater, film and visual arts) and their application to medical education and practice.

4. **health promotion:** 健康促进。根据世界卫生组织（WHO）的建议，健康促进是指促使人们维护和改善其自身健康的过程。Health promotion is the process of enabling people to increase control over, and to improve, their health. It moves beyond a focus on individual behavior towards a wide range of social and environmental interventions.

5. **Hippocrates:** 希波克拉底，公元前 460—前 370；古希腊医生，被称为"医学之父"。希波克拉底订立的医师誓言成为后世医师的道德纲领，传至今日。Hippocrates of Kos was a Greek physician of the classical period who is considered one of the most outstanding figures in the history of medicine. He is traditionally referred to as the "father of medicine" in recognition of his lasting contributions to the field, such as the use of prognosis and clinical observation, the systematic categorization of diseases, and the formulation of humoral theory.

6. **Galen:** 盖伦，129—199（对其卒年存在争议，此仅为一种说法）；古罗马医学家及哲学家。盖伦全名为克劳迪亚斯·盖伦（Claudius Galenus），也被称作"佩加蒙的盖伦"（Galen of Pergamon）。其医学理论与希波克拉底相近，对西方医学影响巨大。Galen was a Greek physician, surgeon and philosopher in the Roman Empire. Considered to be one of the most accomplished of all medical researchers of

antiquity, Galen influenced the development of various scientific disciplines, including anatomy, physiology, pathology, pharmacology, and neurology, as well as philosophy and logic.

7. **Ibn Sina:** 伊本·西拿，980—1037；其阿拉伯名为阿维森纳（Avicenna），是 11 世纪的大医学家、诗人、哲学家、自然科学家，被称为"世界医学之父"。Sina was a Persian polymath who is regarded as one of the most significant physicians, astronomers, philosophers, and writers of the Islamic Golden Age. He was a Muslim Peripatetic philosopher influenced by Greek Aristotelian philosophy.

8. **Ambroise Paré:** 安布鲁瓦兹·帕雷，1510—1590；法国外科医生，被誉为"现代外科之父"，因对枪炮火药伤的温和处理和截肢中的结扎动脉止血法而闻名。Paré is considered one of "the fathers of surgery and modern forensic pathology" and a pioneer in surgical techniques and battlefield medicine, especially in the treatment of wounds. He was also an anatomist, a member of the Parisian barber surgeon guild and invented several surgical instruments.

9. **Andreas Vesalius:** 安德烈·维萨里，1514—1564；法国著名的医生、解剖学家，近代人体解剖学的创始人，于 1543 年出版《人体构造》（*De Humani Corporis Fabrica Libri Septem*）一书，与哥白尼齐名，是科学革命的两大代表人物之一。Vesalius was a 16th-century anatomist, physician, and author of one of the most influential books on human anatomy, *De Humani Corporis Fabrica Libri Septem* (*On the Fabric of the Human Body in Seven Books*). He is often referred to as the founder of modern human anatomy.

10. **William Harvey:** 威廉·哈维，1578—1657；英国著名的生理学家和医生，他发现了血液循环的规律，奠定了近代生理科学发展的基础。Harvey was an English physician who made influential contributions in anatomy and physiology. He was the first known physician to describe completely, and in detail, the systemic circulation and properties of blood being pumped to the brain and the rest of the body by the heart.

11. **Edward Jenner:** 爱德华·詹纳，1749—1823；英国医生、医学家、科学家，以研究及推广牛痘疫苗、防止天花而闻名，被称为"免疫学之父"。他为后人的研究打开了通道，促使巴斯德、科赫等人针对其他疾病寻求治疗和免疫的方法。In the West, Jenner is often called the "father of immunology", and his work is said to have "saved more lives than the work of any other human".

12. **John Snow:** 约翰·斯诺，1813—1858；英国麻醉学家、流行病学家，被认为是麻醉医学和公共卫生医学的开拓者。他最早提出预防霍乱的措施，对 1854 年伦敦西部西敏市苏活区霍乱爆发有突出贡献，被认为是流行病学研究的先驱。Snow is considered one of the founders of modern epidemiology, in part because of his work in tracing the source of a cholera outbreak in Soho, London, in 1854, which he curtailed by removing the handle of a water pump. His findings inspired the adoption of anesthesia as well as fundamental changes in the water and waste systems of London, which led to similar changes in other cities, and a significant improvement in general public health around the world.

13. Ignaz Semmelweis: 伊格纳兹·塞麦尔维斯，1818—1865；匈牙利产科医师，证明产褥热是由医生手部不清洁造成的，并率先提出了相关预防措施。Semmelweis is now known as an early pioneer of antiseptic procedures, described as the "savior of mothers".

14. Florence Nightingale: 弗洛伦斯·南丁格尔，1820—1910；英国护士和统计学家。作为世界上第一个真正的女护士，她开创了护理事业。Nightingale came to prominence while serving as a manager and trainer of nurses during the Crimean War, in which she organized care for wounded soldiers at Constantinople. She gave nursing a favorable reputation and became an icon of Victorian culture, especially in the persona of "The Lady with the Lamp" making rounds of wounded soldiers at night. Recent commentators have asserted that Nightingale's Crimean War achievements were exaggerated by the media at the time, but critics agree on the importance of her later work in professionalizing nursing roles for women.

15. Joseph Lister: 约瑟夫·李斯特，1827—1912；英国外科医师、外科消毒法的创始人及推广者。Lister promoted the idea of sterile surgery while working as a surgeon at the Glasgow Royal Infirmary by successfully introducing phenol (then known as carbolic acid) to sterilize surgical instruments, the patients' skin, sutures and the surgeons' hands. His work led to a reduction in post-operative infections and made surgery safer for patients, distinguishing him as the "father of modern surgery".

16. Louis Pasteur: 路易斯·巴斯德，1822—1895；法国微生物家、化学家，因发现疫苗接种、微生物发酵原理及巴氏杀菌法而闻名，被誉为"细菌学之父"和"微生物学之父"（与罗伯特·科赫并称）。Pasteur's research in chemistry led to remarkable breakthroughs in the understanding of the causes and preventions of diseases, which laid down the foundations of hygiene, public health and much of modern medicine.

17. Robert Koch: 罗伯特·科赫，1843—1910；德国医生、微生物学家，是结核病、霍乱和炭疽等传染病病原体的发现者，也是现代细菌学的主要创始人之一，被称为"微生物学之父"（与路易斯·巴斯德并称）。由他提出的"科赫法则"（确定病原体与特定疾病关系的四个通用医学原理）目前仍在使用，对法则提出之后的流行病学理论产生了重要影响。Koch was awarded the Nobel Prize in Physiology or Medicine in 1905 "for his investigations and discoveries in relation to tuberculosis".

18. **Alexander Fleming:** 亚历山大·弗莱明，1881—1955；英国细菌学家、生物化学家、微生物学家，世界上第一种广泛有效的抗生素——青霉素的发明者，于 1945 年荣获诺贝尔生理学或医学奖。Fleming also discovered and named lysozyme, an antibacterial enzyme found in tears and saliva.

Post-reading Activities

I **Speaking Practice: Group Discussion**

Directions: *Please discuss the following questions in small groups. After your discussion, please share your opinions with the whole class.*

1. Based on your reading, what do you know about the history of medicine? How does it contribute to medical students' understanding of medicine?

2. Do you know any Chinese scientists and doctors who made great contributions to the development of medical sciences?

3. What do you think of the oil painting *The Agnew Clinic*?

II **Speaking Practice: Oral Presentation**

Directions: *The following historical figures have made great contributions to the development of medical sciences. Choose one figure and search for more information on the Internet. Then give an oral presentation to introduce the biography and achievements of the figure to the whole class.*

Hippocrates	*Galen*	*Ibn Sina*	*Ambroise Paré*
Andreas Vesalius	*William Harvey*	*Edward Jenner*	*John Snow*
Ignaz Semmelweis	*Joseph Lister*	*Louis Pasteur*	*Robert Koch*
Alexander Fleming			

Part 2 Thematic Reading

The First Heart Transplant①

Before the 1960s, severe **coronary** artery disease and **congestive** heart failure **spelled** a death sentence for patients. Then in 1967, South African surgeon Christiaan Barnard transplanted a heart from a human donor to a critically ill patient, **heralding** a new era in transplant surgery.

The first slow steps toward successful **transplantation**[1] began in the 1890s, when skin **grafts** using the patient's own tissue were successfully carried out; but those using donor skin, for example from **corpses**, had little success. An attempt to transplant a donor **pancreas** in 1894 also failed. Doctors did not as yet understand the role of the **immune** system in accepting donor organs.

Another **prerequisite** for the complex surgery needed to remove diseased organs and replace them with healthy donated ones, was the ability to perform **vascular suturing**, that is, sew back torn or severed blood **vessels**. This procedure was established by French surgeon Alexis Carrel from 1901 to 1910.

First Transplants

The first transplantation attempts were carried out on dogs, starting with their

---

New Expressions

transplant /ˈtrænzplænt/ *n.*（器官等的）移植	**immune** /ɪˈmjuːn/ *adj.* 有免疫力的
coronary /ˈkɔːrəneri/ *adj.* 冠状动脉的	**prerequisite** /ˌpriːˈrekwəzɪt/ *n.* 先决条件；前提；必备条件
congestive /kənˈdʒestɪv/ *adj.* 充血的	**vascular** /ˈvæskjələr/ *adj.* 血管的；脉管的；维管的
spell /spel/ *v.* 招致，意味着（通常指坏事）	
herald /ˈherəld/ *v.* 是（某事）的前兆；预示	**suture** /ˈsuːtʃər/ *v.*（伤口的）缝合；缝线
graft /ɡræft/ *n.* 移植的皮肤（或骨骼等）；移植	**vessel** /ˈvesl/ *n.*（人或动物的）血管，脉管
corpse /kɔːrps/ *n.* 尸体；（尤指人的）死尸，尸首	
pancreas /ˈpæŋkriəs/ *n.* 胰；胰腺	

---

① The text is adapted from the following source: Parker, S. et al. 2016. *Medicine: The Definitive Illustrated History*. London: DK Publishing.

 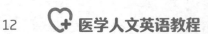

kidneys. The earliest successful **canine** heart transplant was carried out by Norman Lumway and Richard Lower at Stanford, California, in 1959. They used a technique of **topical hypothermia**, in which the donor heart was frozen outside the body, preserving its functions for several hours while surgery was carried out. In 1954, the science of transplantation took a major step forward with the first successful human kidney transplant—between **identical** twins. **Rejection**—when the **recipient**'s immune system attacks a donor organ because it recognizes it as foreign tissue—was a danger, but in this case it was low as the donor and the recipient were genetically identical, and the kidney recipient lived for nine years. In general, the survival rate was much lower because rejection was common. The only way to prevent it was by **massive irradiation** with X-rays to **suppress** the recipient's immune system. In 1959, the first **immunosuppressant** drugs—which **dampen** down the body's immune system—were developed by British surgeon Roy Calne, and survival rates soon improved. These drugs, as well as **refinements** to the heart-lung machines that could take over the function of those organs during surgery, made heart transplants **feasible**. However, **ethical** concerns delayed surgeons from performing the operation for several years.

The Big Leap

On December 3, 1967, Christiaan Barnard, a South African surgeon at Groote Schuur Hospital in Cape Town, successfully transplanted a heart from a donor—a 24-year-old woman who had died in a traffic accident—into the body of 54-year-old Louis Washkansky, who was suffering from a **terminal** heart disease. The operation took nearly five hours: The surgeons first removed Washkansky's diseased heart, and

New Expressions	
kidney /ˈkɪdni/ *n.* 肾；肾脏	**immunosuppressant** /ˌɪmjunousəˈpresnt/ *n.* 免疫抑制剂
canine /ˈkeɪnaɪn/ *adj.* 犬的	
topical /ˈtɑːpɪkl/ *adj.* （身体）局部的	**dampen** /ˈdæmpən/ *v.* 抑制，控制，减弱（感情、反应等）
hypothermia /ˌhaɪpəˈθɜːrmiə/ *n.* 低体温	
identical /aɪˈdentɪkl/ *adj.* 完全同样的；相同的	**refinement** /rɪˈfaɪnmənt/ *n.* （精细的）改进，改善
rejection /rɪˈdʒekʃn/ *n.* 排斥，排异（移植的器官）	**feasible** /ˈfiːzəbl/ *adj.* 可行的；行得通的
recipient /rɪˈsɪpiənt/ *n.* 受方；接受者	**ethical** /ˈeθɪkl/ *adj.* （有关）道德的，伦理的
massive /ˈmæsɪv/ *adj.* 巨大的；非常严重的	**leap** /liːp/ *n.* 跳越；跳跃；跳高
irradiation /ɪˌreɪdiˈeɪʃn/ *n.* 放射	**terminal** /ˈtɜːrmɪnl/ *adj.* （疾病）晚期的，不治的，致命的
suppress /səˈpres/ *v.* 压制；阻止；抑制	

then carefully sutured the blood vessels in his chest to the donor organ. The new heart failed to beat at first, but it was shocked into life with a **defibrillator**[2]. The operation had worked, but 19 days later Washkansky **succumbed** to **pneumonia**, **aggravated** by an immune system that had been suppressed to stop organ rejection.

In January 1968, Barnard operated on his second patient, Philip Blaiberg, who lived for 594 days. Surgeons in other countries began conducting heart transplants and by 1971, 180 operations had been performed. However, survival rates remained disappointing. There was a high rate of rejection and the immunosuppressant drugs had severe side effects. In 1976, Belgian immunologist J. F. Borel discovered the immunosuppressant qualities of **cyclosporine**[3]. It had far fewer toxic side effects than previous **antirejection**[4] drugs and was **licensed** for use in transplant surgery in 1983. When tried in heart surgery, survival rates for patients improved and the number of transplant operations rapidly increased, reaching around 3,500 per year by the early 21st century.

Some heart transplant patients have now lived for over 30 years and the 10-year survival rate has reached 65 to 70 percent. A continuing problem is transplant coronary artery disease—the excessive narrowing of arteries where blood vessels are sewn back together during surgery. Resolving this, the most common cause of death after heart transplantation, is one of the most serious challenges faced by heart surgeons today.

People living only 150 years ago might well have **undergone bloodletting**[5] as part of a medical treatment, so the fact that today **blood transfusions**[6], **open heart surgery**[7], and heart transplants are conducted with frequency is all the more amazing. While physicians would prefer to teach people to live healthy lifestyles so that heart transplants and heart surgery are unnecessary, the reality is that these medical treatments are going

---

New Expressions

defibrillator /diːˈfɪbrɪleɪtər/ *n.* 除颤器（通过电击心脏控制心肌运动）

pneumonia /nuːˈmoʊniə/ *n.* 肺炎

aggravate /ˈæɡrəveɪt/ *v.* 使严重；使恶化

cyclosporine /ˌsaɪkləˈspɔrən/ *n.* 环孢霉素

antirejection /ˌæntɪrɪˈdʒekʃn/ *adj.* （器官移植）防排斥的

license /ˈlaɪsns/ *v.* 批准；许可

undergo /ˌʌndərˈɡoʊ/ *v.* 经历，经受（变化、不快的事等）

bloodletting /ˈblʌdletɪŋ/ *n.* 放血疗法

transfusion /trænsˈfjuːʒn/ *n.* 输血；输液

to continue to be needed. Advances in fixing a patient's own heart will be a top **priority**, but with the difficulty in finding hearts available to transplant, the most promising **frontier** may be in the creation of **miniature artificial** hearts.

New Expressions	
priority /praɪˈɒrəti/ *n.* 优先事项；最重要的事；首要事情	**miniature** /ˈmɪnətʃər/ *adj.* 很小的；微型的；小型的
frontier /frʌnˈtɪr/ *n.* （学科或活动的）尖端，边缘	**artificial** /ˌɑːrtɪˈfɪʃl/ *adj.* 人工的；人造的；假的

Notes

1. **transplantation**: 移植。移植包括细胞、组织或器官的移植，分为同种移植和异种移植。Organs and/or tissues that are transplanted within the same person's body are called autografts. Transplants that are recently performed between two subjects of the same species are called allografts. Allografts can either be from a living or cadaveric source.

2. **defibrillator**: 除颤器。除颤器是向心脏发送电脉冲或电击以恢复正常心跳的设备，用于预防或纠正心律失常，即心跳过慢或过快的不均匀现象。如果心脏突然停止，除颤器也可以帮助它再次跳动。Defibrillators are devices that send an electric pulse or shock to the heart to restore a normal heartbeat. They are used to prevent or correct an arrhythmia, an uneven heartbeat that is too slow or too fast. If the heart suddenly stops, defibrillators can also help it beat again.

3. **cyclosporine**: 环孢霉素。环孢霉素主要用于肝、肾及心脏移植的抗排异反应，可与肾上腺皮质激素同用，也可用于一些免疫性疾病的治疗。Cyclosporine is indicated to treat and prevent graft-versus-host disease in bone marrow transplantation and to prevent rejection of kidney, heart, and liver transplants.

4. **antirejection**: 抗排斥药，也叫免疫抑制剂（immunosuppressant）。Immunosuppressants are drugs or medicines that lower the body's ability to reject a transplanted organ. Another term for these drugs is antirejection drugs. There are two types of immunosuppressants: induction drugs and powerful antirejection medicine used at the time of transplant.

5. **bloodletting**: 放血。放血是将人的血液放出，来治疗、预防或者诊断疾病的替代医学疗法。放血在西方和中东的理论基础是古代医学的体液学说系统。该系统认为如果体液在人体内失去平衡，则会导致疾病，所以人体会适时释放出多余的体液。放血是自古代至近代外科医生最常使用的治疗手段，在欧洲，放血疗法甚至持续到19世纪末。Bloodletting is the withdrawal of blood from a patient to prevent or cure an illness or a disease. Bloodletting, whether by a physician or by leeches, was based on an ancient system of medicine in which blood and other bodily fluids were regarded as "humors" that had to remain in proper balance to maintain health. It is claimed to have been the most common medical practice performed by surgeons from antiquity until the late 19th century, a span of over 2,000 years.

6. **blood transfusions**: 输血。输血是一种治疗措施，被认为是一种支持性与代偿性的疗法，以替代血液中丢失的成分。A blood transfusion provides blood or blood components if the patient lost blood due to an injury, during surgery or certain medical conditions that affect blood or its components. The blood typically comes from donors. Blood banks and health care providers ensure transfusions are a safe, low risk treatment.

7. **open heart surgery**: 心脏外科手术。心脏外科手术是外科医生在病人胸部开一个大切口以打开胸腔并对其心脏进行的手术。Open heart surgery is any type of surgery where the chest is cut open and surgery is performed on the muscles, valves, or arteries of the heart. Open heart surgery is sometimes called traditional heart surgery. Today, many new heart procedures can be performed with only small incisions, not wide openings. Therefore, the term "open heart surgery" can be misleading.

Post-reading Activities

I Language Building-up

Task 1 Extensive Vocabulary Enlargement

Directions: *The following words are taken from the text. Please follow the three-step learning in this part and build up your own Extensive Vocabulary Chart.*

Step 1. Read through the words and underline them in the text. Circle the ones that are particularly new to you. Look up the words in the dictionary and put the equivalent Chinese translation in the chart on the next page.

Step 2. While you go back to the text, please feel free to put any other words into the blanks provided in the extra lines in the chart.

Extensive Vocabulary Chart				
coronary	congestive	graft	pancreas	vascular
suture	kidney	canine	hypothermia	irradiation
immunosuppressant	dampen	defibrillator	pneumonia	cyclosporine
antirejection	transfusion	frontier	miniature	artificial

Step 3. Please group the above words based on their parts of speech and meanings.

Nouns	
Verbs	
Adjectives	
Adverbs and Prepositions	
Medical Terminology	
Terminology in Other Fields	

Directions: *The following 10 words are chosen from the text. They will form the intensive vocabulary in this unit. For intensive vocabulary, you are supposed to be able to explain them in English and use them in sentence and discourse constructions.*

Step 1.　Please read through the words and be familiar with their Chinese and English definitions. Recall where and how they are used in the text.

No.	Word	Translation	Definition	Status
			Intensive Vocabulary Chart	
1	transplant	（器官等的）移植	*n.* a medical operation in which a damaged organ, etc. is replaced with one from another person	☆☆☆☆☆
2	herald	是（某事）的前兆；预示	*v.* to be a sign that sth. is going to happen	☆☆☆☆☆
3	identical	完全同样的；相同的	*adj.* similar in every detail	☆☆☆☆☆
4	suppress	压制；阻止；抑制	*v.* to prevent sth. from growing, developing, or continuing	☆☆☆☆☆
5	refinement	（精细的）改进，改善	*n.* a small change to sth. that improves it	☆☆☆☆☆
6	ethical	（有关）道德的；伦理的	*adj.* connected with beliefs and principles about what is right and wrong	☆☆☆☆☆
7	leap	跳越；跳跃；跳高	*n.* a long or high jump	☆☆☆☆☆
8	terminal	（疾病）晚期的；不治的；致命的	*adj.* (of an illness or a disease) that cannot be cured and will lead to death, often slowly	☆☆☆☆☆
9	aggravate	使严重；使恶化	*v.* to make an illness or a bad or unpleasant situation worse	☆☆☆☆☆
10	license	批准；许可	*v.* to give sb. official permission to do, own, or use sth.	☆☆☆☆☆

Step 2.　Please tick the status for each word based on your own situation. If one word is very new or difficult for you, please tick five stars. Likewise, if one word is comparatively easy for you and you don't have to spend too much time on reading and learning it, then tick one star. The number of stars represents the difficulty of commanding a word in your eyes.

Step 3. Please complete the following 10 sentences by choosing appropriate words from the Intensive Vocabulary Chart. Please change the forms of the words where necessary.

1. They didn't realize his cancer was _____.
   他们并未意识到他的癌症已经处于晚期。

2. Several companies have been _____ to sell these products.
   一些公司获得了这些产品的销售许可。

3. Few people successfully make the _____ from television to the movies.
   很少有人成功地从电视业转向电影业。

4. The president's speech _____ a new era in foreign policy.
   总统的演说预示着一个外交政策新时代的开始。

5. The doctor has prescribed some drugs to _____ her appetite.
   医生给她开了一些抑制食欲的药。

6. Military intervention will only _____ the conflict even further.
   军事介入只会使冲突加剧。

7. The two pictures are similar, although not _____.
   这两幅画虽然很相似，但不完全相同。

8. This is a medical procedure that most people believe to be _____.
   这是一项大多数人认为合乎伦理准则的医学程序。

9. He had a liver _____ last year.
   他去年做了一个肝脏移植手术。

10. These _____ have increased the machine's accuracy by 25 percent.
    经过这些改进，机器的准确率提高了25%。

Task 3　Expressions and Sentences

Directions: *The following sentences are taken from the text. In each sentence, there are one or two phrases being underlined. Please refer to the dictionary and write down the explanation of the phrases in the line entitled "Meaning Exploration". After that, please choose one phrase and make a sentence with it. Write the sentence in the line entitled "Sentence Making".*

Original Sentence	Before the 1960s, severe coronary artery disease and congestive heart failure spelled a death sentence for patients.
Meaning Exploration	*spell a death sentence*: to announce that death is unavoidably coming
Sentence Making	With the development of science and technology, the diagnosis of cancer no longer *spells a death sentence* for patients.

Sentence 1

Original Sentence	Then in 1967, South African surgeon Christiaan Barnard transplanted a heart from a human donor to a critically ill patient, heralding a new era in transplant surgery.
Meaning Exploration	*herald a new era:*
Sentence Making	

Sentence 2

Original Sentence	Another prerequisite for the complex surgery needed to remove diseased organs and replace them with healthy donated ones, was the ability to perform vascular suturing, that is, sew back torn or severed blood vessels.
Meaning Exploration	*replace A with B:*
Sentence Making	

Sentence 3

Original Sentence	The operation had worked, but 19 days later Washkansky succumbed to pneumonia, aggravated by an immune system that had been suppressed to stop organ rejection.
Meaning Exploration	*(be) aggravated by:* *(be) suppressed to:*
Sentence Making	

Sentence 4

Original Sentence	These drugs, as well as refinements to the heart-lung machines that could take over the function of those organs during surgery, made heart transplants feasible.
Meaning Exploration	*take over the function of:* *make (sth.) feasible:*
Sentence Making	

Sentence 5

Original Sentence	Advances in fixing a patient's own heart will be a top priority, but with the difficulty in finding hearts available to transplant, the most promising frontier may be in the creation of miniature artificial hearts.
Meaning Exploration	*in the creation of:*
Sentence Making	

II Critical Reading and Thinking

Task 1   Overview and Comprehension

Directions: *The text can be divided into three small parts, namely introduction, first transplants, and the big leap. Please write down the main information provided in each part based on your reading.*

Reading Notes	
Introduction	
First Transplants	
The Big Leap	

Directions: *After reading, please reflect on the theme of the text. Work in groups and share your opinions on the following questions with other group members.*

1. What is known about the transplantation practices in the 1890s and what were the major drawbacks at that time?

2. What do you know about the first attempts on transplantation practices? Please describe the key techniques used and the process of surgery based on your reading.

3. What are the main challenges doctors faced in their early attempts to transplant organs on human bodies in the modern era?

4. What do you know about the first successful heart transplantation on human body? Please describe the details.

5. What are the main challenges of heart transplantation doctors have to face nowadays?

Part 3 Extended Reading

Nursing①

Although nursing is one of the oldest medical occupations, it has not always had a good reputation. It took the influence of one extraordinary woman—Florence Nightingale—to transform nurses from uneducated "ward maids" to the academically qualified, skilled professionals that we know today.

In Europe during the **medieval period**[1], hospitals were usually attached to religious institutions, such as monasteries and **convents**, with patients nursed by monks and nuns. However, in the 16th century many hospitals were shut down as a result of **the Protestant reformation**[2]. With the growth of **industrialization** in the 18th century, new **secular** hospitals were founded. During this period, sometimes termed the "Dark Ages of Nursing", the quality of care was frequently **dire**—nurses tended to be recovering patients, or hired men and women who could not read or write and often drawn from the poorhouses. Nurses gained a reputation for **ignorance**, drunkenness, and misbehavior.

The push for nursing reform in Europe began in the 19th century, largely **instigated** by the Christian community. Many visitors to Germany were impressed by the work of pastor **Theodor Fliedner**[3], who opened a hospital on the **Rhine**[4] in 1836. Nurses were

New Expressions	
occupation /ˌɑːkjuˈpeɪʃn/ n. 工作；职业	**industrialization** /ɪnˌdʌstriələˈzeɪʃn/ n. 工业化
reputation /ˌrepjuˈteɪʃn/ n. 名誉；名声	**secular** /ˈsekjələr/ adj. 现世的；世俗的；非宗教的
transform /trænsˈfɔːrm/ v. 使改变外观（或性质）；使改观	**dire** /ˈdaɪər/ adj. 极糟的；极差的
professional /prəˈfeʃənl/ n. 专门人员；专业人士；专家	**ignorance** /ˈɪɡnərəns/ n. 无知
convent /ˈkɑːnvent/ n. 女隐修院；女修道院	**instigate** /ˈɪnstɪɡeɪt/ v. 使（正式）开始；使发生

---

① The text is adapted from the following source: Parker, S. et al. 2016. *Medicine: The Definitive Illustrated History*. London: DK Publishing.

given simple clinical instruction and studied pharmacy—the practice of preparing and **dispensing** drugs. The nursing course was quite advanced for its time, and Fliedner's most famous student—Florence Nightingale—spent three months at his hospital in 1851. By the mid-19th century, the concept of women being trained to nurse was well established.

Nurses Go to War

The **advent** of the **Crimean War**[5] (1853—1856) transformed nursing. **Cholera**[6] spread rapidly in the British army camp, and surgeons had to perform major operations and **amputations** without light, **anesthetics**, or even **bandages**. When the British press reported that the wounded and the sick were not being properly cared for, the government responded by sending female nurses abroad to tend to the **casualties**. Florence Nightingale was appointed as the "**Superintendent** of the Female Nursing **Establishment** of the English General Hospitals in Türkiye"—a powerful position that gathered huge attention.

Nightingale enforced a strict **code** of discipline, discouraging nurses from **fraternizing** with the patients and doctors, as well as promoting **hygiene**, **sobriety** at all times, and good manners. Nightingale and her small band of nurses were a great inspiration to women, showing that war was no longer a male **preserve**. When the **American Civil War**[7] broke out in 1861, the **Sanitary Commission**[8]—a forerunner to the **Red Cross**[9]—was founded. Armed with the knowledge of good hygiene practices from the Crimean War, it **recruited** a large number of nurses.

New Expressions	
dispense /dɪ'spens/ v. 配（药）；发（药）	**establishment** /ɪ'stæblɪʃmənt/ n. 机构；大型机关；企业；旅馆
advent /'ædvent/ n.（重要事件、人物、发明等的）出现，到来	**code** /koʊd/ n. 道德准则；行为规范
amputation /ˌæmpju'teɪʃn/ n. 截（肢）	**fraternize** /'frætərnaɪz/ v.（尤指与不该亲善者）亲善
anesthetic /ˌænəs'θetɪk/ n. 麻醉药；麻醉剂	**hygiene** /'haɪdʒiːn/ n. 卫生
bandage /'bændɪdʒ/ n. 绷带	**sobriety** /sə'braɪəti/ n. 未醉；节制；持重；冷静
casualty /'kæʒʊəlti/ n.（战争或事故的）伤员，亡者，遇难者	**preserve** /prɪ'zɜːrv/ n.（某人或群体活动、工作等的）专门领域
superintendent /ˌsuːpərɪn'tendənt/ n. 主管人；负责人；监管人；监督人	**recruit** /rɪ'kruːt/ v. 吸收（新成员）；征募（新兵）

医学人文英语教程

A Modern Profession

Until World War I the Nightingale legacy prevailed. Nurses were seen as the **guardians** of hygiene, the **dispensers** of **compassion**, and the center of calm amid the chaos of the hospital. However, the nurses' actual duties were rather vaguely described. During World War I, the boundaries between medicine and nursing broke down. As doctors struggled to cope with emergency surgery, trained nursing staff took on duties that would not normally fall to them, including **triage**, the **administration** of **saline** drips and **intravenous** injections, and the dispensing of **narcotic** drugs. The nursing staff were also responsible for **implementing** many of the new developments aimed at combating infection and passing on their knowledge to volunteers from the **Red Cross's Voluntary Aid Detachments (VADs)**[10], which were set up to provide **supplementary first aid**[11] and nursing to the medical service in wartime. In addition, nurses had to cope with the effects of new wartime technology—for example, learning how to use **oxygen cylinders** for soldiers with lungs filled with mustard gas, and applying **sodium bicarbonate**[12] to their blinded eyes.

World Wars I and II emphasized the growing need for fully trained, well-educated nurses, and today many countries **demand** that nurses have a university degree. From an occupation of the poor and **illiterate**, nursing has **evolved** to become one of the most important professions within the health care industry.

New Expressions

guardian /ˈgɑːrdiən/ *n.* 保护者；守卫者；保卫者

dispenser /dɪˈspensər/ *n.* 药剂师；配药师

compassion /kəmˈpæʃn/ *n.* 同情；怜悯

triage /triːˈɑːʒ/ *n.* 患者鉴别分类；伤员鉴别分类；治疗类选法

administration /ədˌmɪnɪˈstreɪʃn/ *n.*（药物的）施用

saline /ˈseɪliːn/ *n.* 盐水

intravenous /ˌɪntrəˈviːnəs/ *adj.* 注入静脉的；静脉内的

narcotic /nɑːrˈkɑːtɪk/ *adj.* 致幻的；麻醉的

implement /ˈɪmplɪment/ *v.* 使生效；贯彻；执行；实施

supplementary /ˌsʌplɪˈmentri/ *adj.* 增补性的；补充性的；额外的；外加的

cylinder /ˈsɪlɪndər/ *n.*（尤指用作容器的）圆筒状物

oxygen cylinder 氧气瓶

sodium /ˈsoʊdiəm/ *n.* 钠

bicarbonate /baɪˈkɑːrbənət/ *n.* 碳酸氢盐

sodium bicarbonate 碳酸氢钠

demand /dɪˈmænd/ *v.* 强烈要求

illiterate /ɪˈlɪtərət/ *adj.* 不会读写的；不识字的；文盲的

evolve /iˈvɑːlv/ *v.*（使）逐渐形成；逐步发展；逐渐演变

Florence Nightingale

British Nurse

Born into a wealthy English family, Florence Nightingale reformed the profession of nursing. A woman of very strong will, her **tireless** work caring for soldiers during the Crimean War established her as "The Lady with the Lamp". Her reforms led to a **dramatic reduction** in deaths. She founded a training school for nurses at St. Thomas' Hospital, London, in 1860, and helped promote nursing as a respectable career for women.

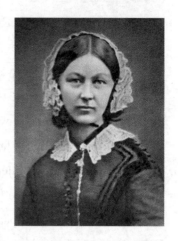

New Expressions

tireless /'taɪərləs/ *adj.* 不知疲倦的；不觉疲劳的；精力充沛的

dramatic /drə'mætɪk/ *adj.* 突然的；巨大的；令人吃惊的

reduction /rɪ'dʌkʃn/ *n.* 减少；缩小；降低

Notes

1. **medieval period:** 中世纪时期。中世纪时期是欧洲历史三大传统划分的中间时期（三段时期分别为古典时代、中世纪和近现代），指西罗马帝国灭亡到东罗马帝国灭亡的时期，大概为公元 5 世纪至 15 世纪。The Middle Ages or medieval period lasted approximately from the 5th to the 15th century. It began with the fall of the Western Roman Empire and transitioned into the Renaissance and the Age of Discovery. The Late Middle Ages was marked by difficulties and calamities including famine, plague, and war, which significantly diminished the population of Europe; between 1347 and 1350, the Black Death killed about a third of Europeans.

2. **the Protestant reformation:** 新教改革。这是一场在 16 世纪席卷欧洲的宗教改革运动，它对天主教会，尤其是对教皇权威提出了宗教和政治挑战。新教改革之后，西方教会分裂为新教会和罗马天主教会。It is also considered to be one of the events that signified the end of the Middle Ages and the beginning of the early modern period in Europe.

3. **Theodor Fliedner:** 西奥多·弗利德纳，1800—1864；德国新教牧师、社会改革者、

福音派护士教育学院的创始人，在护理方面的工作对弗洛伦斯·南丁格尔产生了很大影响。To better support and teach Kaiserwerth's children, Fliedner founded a school in 1835 which became the venue for a women teachers' seminar.

4. **Rhine:** 莱茵地区。莱茵地区是指莱茵河流经的地区。本文所提到的弗利德纳（见 Note 3）所建立的医院位于德国城市杜塞尔多夫的凯泽斯韦尔特，毗邻莱茵河畔。The Rhine is a vital navigable waterway bringing trade and goods deep inland in Europe.

5. **Crimean War:** 克里米亚战争。这是于 1853—1856 年在欧洲爆发的一场战争。英国女护士南丁格尔在这场战争中赴前线护理伤病员，使伤病员死亡率下降，由此促进了战地医疗的改善和南丁格尔护理制度的诞生。The Crimean War was a military conflict fought from October 1853 to February 1856 in which Russia lost to an alliance of France, the Ottoman Empire, the United Kingdom, and Piedmont-Sardinia.

6. **Cholera:** 霍乱。霍乱是由霍乱弧菌的某些致病株感染小肠而导致的急性腹泻疾病。Cholera affects an estimated 3 million–5 million people worldwide and causes 28,800–130,000 deaths a year. Seven large outbreaks have occurred over the last 200 years with millions of deaths.

7. **American Civil War:** 美国内战。美国内战又称南北战争，是美国历史上最大规模的内战，参战双方为北方的美利坚合众国（简称"联邦"，Union）和南方的美利坚联盟国（简称"邦联"，Confederate）。The American Civil War (April 12, 1861–April 9, 1865) was a civil war in the United States between the Union (states that remained loyal to the federal union, or "the North") and the Confederate (states that voted to secede, or "the South"). The central cause of the war was the status of slavery, especially the expansion of slavery into territories acquired as a result of the Louisiana Purchase and the Mexican-American War. On the eve of the Civil War, 4 million of the 32 million Americans were enslaved black people, almost all in the South.

8. **Sanitary Commission:** 美国卫生委员会。其全称为 United States Sanitary Commission (USSC)，是根据联邦立法于 1861 年 6 月 18 日成立的私人救济机构，旨在支持美国内战期间美国陆军（联邦/北方/联合军）的伤病士兵。The United States Sanitary Commission was the only civilian-run organization recognized by the federal government, served as the focal point for civilian assistance to the military.

9. **Red Cross:** 红十字会。红十字会是国际性的人道主义组织，致力于保护人的生命和健康，保障人类尊严，减轻人类疾苦，不因国籍、种族、宗教信仰、阶级和政治观念而加以任何歧视。Established in 1863, the International Committee of the Red Cross operates worldwide, helping people affected by conflict and armed violence and promoting the laws that protect victims of war.

10. **Red Cross's Voluntary Aid Detachments (VADs)**: 红十字会自愿救助队。Voluntary Aid Detachment members themselves came to be known simply as "VADs". Made up of men and women, the VADs carried out a range of voluntary positions including nursing, transport duties, and the organization of rest stations, working parties and auxiliary hospitals.

11. **first aid**: 急救。First aid is the first and immediate assistance given to any person suffering from either a minor or serious illness or injury, with care provided to preserve life, prevent the condition from worsening, or to promote recovery.

12. **sodium bicarbonate**: 碳酸氢钠。战争中常用的一些毒气，如芥子气、路易氏气等，会对眼睛造成损害。其急救方法之一就是用 2% 的碳酸氢钠冲洗眼睛。Sodium bicarbonate is a chemical compound with the formula $NaHCO_3$. It is a chemical in the form of a white powder that dissolves and is used in baking to make cakes and in making fizzy drinks and some medicines.

Post-reading Activities

I **Speaking Practice: Interview**

Directions: *Please work in pairs. Imagine one of you is an interviewee, a professor of history of nursing, and the other is an interviewer who interviews the professor about the history of nursing. Please design three interview questions and take turns to be the interviewer and the interviewee.*

Interview questions:

1. _____

2. _____

3. _____

II Reflective Writing Practice: Short Essay

Directions: *Nursing is one of the oldest medical occupations in the world, but its important role has not been fully recognized. Please think about the role of nurses in delivering quality health care to patients and write a reflective essay entitled "Nursing in My Eyes". The word limit is suggested to be 150–200 words.*

Unit 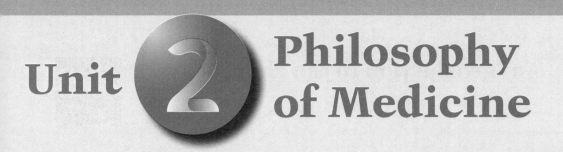 Philosophy of Medicine

> *Wherever the art of medicine is loved, there is also a love of humanity.*
>
> —Hippocrates

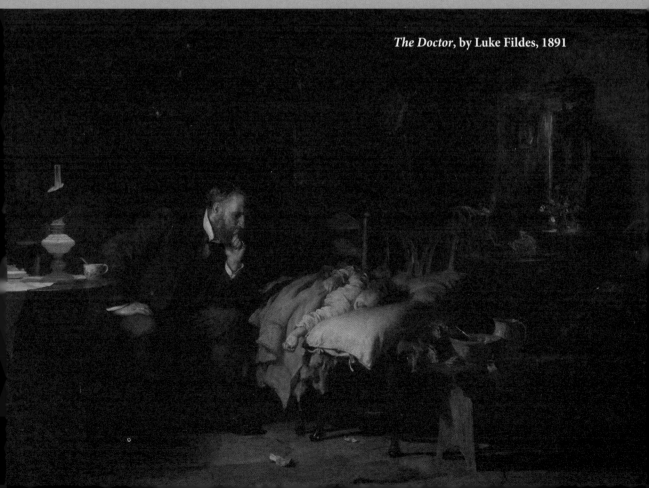

The Doctor, by Luke Fildes, 1891

Part 1 Academic Horizon

An Introduction to the Philosophy of Medicine①

Philosophy of medicine is a field that seeks to explore fundamental issues in theory, research, and practice within the health sciences, particularly **metaphysical** and **epistemological** topics. Its historic roots arguably **date back to** ancient times, to the **Hippocratic corpus**[1] among other sources, and there have been extended scholarly discussions on key concepts in the philosophy of medicine since at least the 1800s.

Philosophy of medicine has become a vibrant intellectual **landscape**. Medicine is, of course, a hugely important practice in our society. Two of the main aims of medicine are to care and to cure. That sounds simple. But in the **pursuit** of these aims, medicine relies on concepts, theories, inferences, and policies that are complicated and **controversial**.

What makes a problem philosophical? Philosophical problems are those for which there exist multiple **compelling** and competing views, and which cannot be answered straightforwardly by **empirical** means. There are many problems like this in various **domains** of life, such as ethics, religion, and politics. Philosophy of medicine is the study

---

New Expressions	
metaphysical /ˌmetəˈfɪzɪkl/ *adj.* 形而上学的	**controversial** /ˌkɑːntrəˈvɜːrʃl/ *adj.* 引起争论的；有争议的
epistemological /ɪˌpɪstəməˈlɑdʒəkəl/ *adj.* 认识论的	**compelling** /kəmˈpelɪŋ/ *adj.* 令人信服的
date back to 可追溯到；始于（某时期）	**empirical** /ɪmˈpɪrɪkl/ *adj.* 以实验（或经验）为依据的；经验主义的
landscape /ˈlændskeɪp/ *n.*（陆上，尤指乡村的）风景，景色	**domain** /douˈmeɪn/ *n.*（知识、活动的）领域，范围，范畴
pursuit /pərˈsuːt/ *n.* 追求；寻找	

---

① The text is adapted from the following sources: Stegenga, J. 2018. *Care and Cure: An Introduction to Philosophy of Medicine*. Chicago: University of Chicago Press.

Reiss, J. & Ankeny, R. A. 2016. Philosophy of medicine. *Stanford Encyclopedia of Philosophy*. Retrieved October 20, 2022, from Stanford Encyclopedia of Philosophy website.

of epistemological, metaphysical, and logical aspects of medicine, with occasional forays into historical, sociological, and political aspects of medicine.

The nature of medicine raises fundamental questions about explanation, causation, knowledge, and ontology—questions that are central to philosophy as well as medicine. Does being healthy involve merely the absence of disease, or does being healthy require some other positive factors? Is a disease simply an abnormal physiological state, or is a disease a state that has an evaluative component? Is social anxiety disorder a genuine disease? What sort of evidence is required to justify causal inferences about the effectiveness of medical interventions? Is medicine good at achieving its aims of caring and curing—are most mainstream medical interventions effective? Is homeopathy[2] effective? Does psychiatry aim to care for patients with mental illnesses, or rather does psychiatry aim to control feelings and behaviors that do not fit well with modern society? Should medical innovations be protected by patent, or should such innovations be contributions to the common good, unprotected by intellectual property laws?

Many of these questions are interrelated. For example, consider this seemingly straightforward question: Are antidepressants effective for treating depression? Of course, this is in part an empirical question, and so answering the question requires a compelling view about what sort of evidence is required to answer such questions. Since that evidence comes out of a thorny social, legal, and financial nexus, a full understanding of an answer to this question requires insight into that nexus. Since

New Expressions	
foray /'fɔːreɪ/ *n.*（改变职业、活动的）尝试	**intervention** /ˌɪntər'venʃn/ *n.* 介入；干涉；干预
causation /kɔː'zeɪʃn/ *n.* 诱因；起因；原因	**mainstream** /'meɪnstriːm/ *adj.* 主流的
ontology /ɑːn'tɑːlədʒi/ *n.* 本体论；存在论	**homeopathy** /ˌhoʊmi'ɑːpəθi/ *n.* 顺势疗法
merely /'mɪrli/ *adv.* 仅仅；只不过	**psychiatry** /saɪ'kaɪətri/ *n.* 精神病学；精神病治疗
absence /'æbsəns/ *n.* 不存在；缺乏	**patent** /'pætnt/ *n.* 专利权；专利证书
abnormal /æb'nɔːrml/ *adj.* 不正常的；反常的；变态的；畸形的	**interrelated** /ˌɪntərɪ'leɪtɪd/ *adj.* 相互关联的
physiological /ˌfɪziə'lɑːdʒɪkl/ *adj.* 生理的	**antidepressant** /ˌæntidɪ'presnt/ *n.* 抗抑郁药；抗抑郁剂
evaluative /ɪ'væljuətɪv/ *adj.* 评估的	**thorny** /'θɔːrni/ *adj.* 棘手的；麻烦的；引起争议的
component /kəm'poʊnənt/ *n.* 组成部分；成分；部件	**nexus** /'neksəs/ *n.*（错综复杂的）关系，连接，联系
disorder /dɪs'ɔːrdər/ *n.* 失调；紊乱；不适；疾病	
genuine /'dʒenjuɪn/ *adj.* 真的；名副其实的	

antidepressants are said to target localized **micro-physiological entities**, answering the question depends on a view about the relationship between the experiences of people—their feelings and behaviors and symptoms—and the activities of chemicals. Since the question is about a disease category that many people consider to be poorly understood and indeed controversial, properly understanding the question requires insight into the general nature of health and disease.

Medicine is a vast enterprise. Clinical medicine is the familiar practice of physicians and other health care workers attempting to care for patients in a **multitude** of ways. Clinical research is the study of the efficacy of interventions, but of course medicine relies on more fundamental scientific research (sometimes called **bench science**[3]) **prior to** testing interventions in humans. Medicine has many **subspecialities**, such as internal medicine, surgery, psychiatry, and **epidemiology**. Governmental policies and regulations control medicine. Medical research and clinical practice are guided by numerous intellectual and institutional movements, such as **evidence-based medicine**[4] and **personalized (or "precision") medicine**[5]. Philosophical problems arise in all of these aspects of the wide domain of medicine.

New Expressions	
micro-physiological /ˌmaɪkroʊˌfɪziə'lɑːdʒɪkl/ *adj.* 微生理的	**subspeciality** /'səbˌspeʃiˌæləti/ *n.* 分科；附属专业
entity /'entəti/ *n.* 独立存在物；实体	**epidemiology** /ˌepɪˌdiːmi'ɑːlədʒi/ *n.* 流行病学
multitude /'mʌltɪtuːd/ *n.* 众多；大量	**precision** /prɪ'sɪʒn/ *n.* 精确；准确；细致
prior to 在……之前	

Notes

1. **Hippocratic corpus**: 希波克拉底文集。希波克拉底文集包括约 60 篇医学文本，由希波克拉底学派的不同医者撰写而成，大部分文本写于公元前 5 世纪—前 4 世纪，为西方医学实践的建立奠定了基础。The Hippocratic corpus is a collection of around 60 early Ancient Greek medical works strongly associated with the physician Hippocrates and his teachings.

2. **homeopathy**: 顺势疗法。顺势疗法是替代医学的一种，于 1796 年由德国医生塞缪尔·哈内曼提出。A basic belief behind homeopathy is "like cures like". In other

words, something that brings on symptoms in a healthy person can—in a very small dose—treat an illness with similar symptoms. This is meant to trigger the body's natural defenses.

3. bench science: 实验室科学。"bench" 指的是实验室的操作台，实验室科学由此得名。Bench science is scientific research experimentation, usually conducted in a laboratory. The bench alludes to the workbench in a laboratory, upon which equipment would be assembled and operated in the activities of the bench scientist.

4. evidence-based medicine: 循证医学，其缩写为 EBM。循证医学指的是在对个别病人的护理做出决定时，有意识、明确且明智地使用当前的最佳证据的医学诊疗方法。循证医学的目的是整合临床医生的经验、病人的价值观和现有的最佳科学信息，以指导临床管理决策。该术语最初是用来描述一种医学实践的指导方法，旨在改善医生对个别病人的决策。The aim of EBM is to integrate the experience of the clinician, the values of the patient, and the best available scientific information to guide decision-making about clinical management. The term was originally used to describe an approach to teaching the practice of medicine and improving decisions by individual physicians about individual patients.

5. personalized (or "precision") medicine: 个性化（或"精准"）医疗。这是一种新兴的疾病治疗和预防方法，它考虑到每个人在基因、环境和生活方式方面的个体差异，针对特定疾病为病人量身定制治疗或预防计划，包括关于药物使用、降低疾病风险的健康习惯或比平时更早开始筛查疾病的具体建议。Personalized medicine, sometimes known as "precision medicine" is an innovative approach to tailoring disease prevention and treatment that takes into account differences in people's genes, environments, and lifestyles.

Post-reading Activities

I **Speaking Practice: Group Discussion**

Directions: *Please discuss the following questions in small groups. After your discussion, please share your opinions with the whole class.*

1. What is philosophy of medicine?

2. What are the fundamental aims of medicine?

3. What makes a problem philosophical?

4. How can you answer the question "Are antidepressants effective for treating depression?" from the perspective of philosophy of medicine?

Ⅱ Speaking Practice: Oral Presentation

Directions: *According to the text, we know that "The nature of medicine raises fundamental questions about explanation, causation, knowledge, and ontology—questions that are central to philosophy as well as medicine." Please focus on the question "Does being healthy involve merely the absence of disease, or does being healthy require some other positive factors?" and give an oral presentation.*

Part 2 Thematic Reading

Disease and Health[①]

One of the fundamental and most long-standing debates in the philosophy of medicine relates to the basic concepts of health and disease.

It may seem obvious what we mean by such **statements**: People seek treatment from medical professionals when they are feeling unwell, and clinicians treat patients in order to help them restore or **maintain** their health. But people seek advice and assistance from medical professionals for other reasons, such as **pregnancy** which cannot **be construed as** a disease state, and high blood pressure which is **asymptomatic**. Thus the **dividing line** between disease and health is **notoriously** vague, due in part to the wide range of **variations** present in the human population and to debates over whether many concepts of disease are socially constructed. One of the further complicating factors is that both the concepts of health and disease **typically** involve both **descriptive** and **evaluatory** aspects, both in common usage among **lay persons**[1] and members of the medical profession.

Exploring these distinctions remains **epistemologically** and morally important

New Expressions	
statement /'steɪtmənt/ *n.* 声明；陈述；报告	**variation** /ˌveri'eɪʃn/ *n.*（数量、水平等的）变化，变更，变异
maintain /meɪn'teɪn/ *v.* 维持；保持	**typically** /'tɪpɪkli/ *adv.* 通常；一般
pregnancy /'pregnənsi/ *n.* 怀孕；妊娠；孕期	**descriptive** /dɪ'skrɪptɪv/ *adj.* 描写的；叙述的；说明的
be construed as 被理解为	
asymptomatic /ˌeɪsɪmptə'mætɪk/ *adj.* 无症状的	**evaluatory** /ɪ'væljueɪˌtɔːri/ *adj.* 评估的
dividing line （两种事物或思想的）分界线，界限	**epistemologically** /ɪˌpɪstəmə'lɑdʒəkli/ *adv.* 认识论地
notoriously /noʊ'tɔːriəsli/ *adv.* 声名狼藉地；众所周知地	

① The text is adapted from the following sources: Reiss, J. & Ankeny, R. A. 2016. Philosophy of medicine. *Stanford Encyclopedia of Philosophy*. Retrieved November 11, 2022, from Stanford Encyclopedia of Philosophy website.

Marcum, J. A. 2022. Philosophy of medicine. *Internet Encyclopedia of Philosophy*. Retrieved November 11, 2022, from Internet Encyclopedia of Philosophy website.

as these definitions influence when and where people seek medical treatment, and whether society regards them as "ill", including in some health systems whether they are **permitted** to receive treatment. As **Tristram Engelhardt**[2] has argued, the concept of disease acts not only to describe and explain, but also to **enjoin** to action. It **indicates** a state of affairs as **undesirable** and to be overcome.

Hence how we define disease, health, and related concepts is not a matter of mere philosophical or theoretical interest, but **critical** for ethical reasons, particularly to make certain that medicine contributes to people's well-being, and for social reasons, as one's well-being is critically related to whether one can live a good life.

"What is disease?" is a **contentious** question among philosophers of medicine. These philosophers distinguish among four different notions of disease. The first is an **ontological** notion. According to its **proponents**, disease is a **palpable** object or entity whose existence is distinct from that of the diseased patient. For example, disease may be the condition brought on by the infection of a **microorganism**, such as a virus. Critics, who **champion** a physiological notion of disease, argue that **advocates** of the ontological notion confuse the disease condition, which is an abstract notion, with a **concrete** entity like a virus. In other words, proponents of the first notion often combine the disease's condition and cause. Supporters of this second notion argue that disease represents a **deviation** from normal physiological functioning. The best-known **defender** of this notion is **Christopher Boorse**[3], who defines disease as a value-free statistical norm with respect to "species design". Critics who object to this notion, however, cite the **ambiguity** of the term "norm" in terms of a reference class. Instead of a statistical norm,

New Expressions	
permit /pər'mɪt/ *v.* 允许；准许	**palpable** /'pælpəbl/ *adj.* 易于察觉的；可意识到的；明显的
enjoin /ɪn'dʒɔɪn/ *v.* 命令；责令；嘱咐	**microorganism** /ˌmaɪkroʊ'ɔːrɡənɪzəm/ *n.* 微生物
indicate /'ɪndɪkeɪt/ *v.* 表明；标示；显示	**champion** /'tʃæmpiən/ *v.* 为……而斗争；捍卫；声援
undesirable /ˌʌndɪ'zaɪərəbl/ *adj.* 不想要的；不得人心的；易惹麻烦的	**advocate** /'ædvəkət/ *n.* 拥护者；支持者；提倡者
critical /'krɪtɪkl/ *adj.* 极重要的；关键的；至关紧要的	**concrete** /'kɑːŋkriːt/ *adj.* 确实的，具体的（而非想象或猜测的）
contentious /kən'tenʃəs/ *adj.* 可能引起争论的	**deviation** /ˌdiːvi'eɪʃn/ *n.* 背离；偏离；违背
ontological /ˌɑːntə'lɑːdʒɪkl/ *adj.* 存在论的；本体论的；实体论的	**defender** /dɪ'fendər/ *n.* 守卫者；保护人；防御者
proponent /prə'poʊnənt/ *n.* 倡导者；支持者；拥护者	**ambiguity** /ˌæmbɪ'ɡjuːəti/ *n.* 歧义；一语多义

evolutionary biologists propose a notion of disease as a **maladaptive** mechanism, which factors in the organism's biological history. Critics of this third notion claim that disease **manifests** itself, especially clinically, in terms of the individual patient and not a population. A population may be important to epidemiologists but not to **clinicians** who must treat individual patients whose manifestation of a disease and response to **therapy** for that disease may differ from each other significantly. The final notion of disease **addresses** this criticism. The genetic notion claims that disease is the **mutation** in or absence of a gene. Its champions assert that each patient's **genomic constitution** is **unique**. By knowing the genomic constitution, clinicians are able to both diagnose the patient's disease and **tailor** a specific therapeutic **protocol**. Critics of the genetic notion claim that disease, especially its experience, cannot be reduced to **nucleotide sequences**. Instead, it requires a larger notion including social and cultural factors.

"What is health?" is an equally contentious question among philosophers of medicine. The most common notion of health is simply absence of disease. Health, according to proponents of this notion, represents a **default** state as opposed to **pathology**. In other words, if an organism is not sick, then it must be healthy. Unfortunately, this notion does not distinguish between various grades of health or **preconditions** towards illness. For example, as cells responsible for **serotonin** stop producing the **neurotransmitter**, a person is **prone** to depression. Such a person is not as **healthful** as a person who is making sufficient amounts of serotonin. An adequate

---

New Expressions

evolutionary /ˌevəˈluːʃəneri/ *adj.* 进化的；演变的；逐渐发展的

maladaptive /ˌmæləˈdæptɪv/ *adj.* (个体、物种等)不适应的，适应不良的

manifest /ˈmænɪfest/ *v.* 表明；清楚显示(尤指情感、态度或品质)

clinician /klɪˈnɪʃn/ *n.* 临床医师

therapy /ˈθerəpi/ *n.* 治疗；疗法

address /əˈdres/ *v.* 设法解决；处理；对付

mutation /mjuːˈteɪʃn/ *n.* (生物物种的)变异，突变

genomic /dʒəˈnoumɪk/ *adj.* 染色体组的

constitution /ˌkɑːnstəˈtuːʃn/ *n.* 构成；构造

unique /juˈniːk/ *adj.* 唯一的；独一无二的

tailor /ˈteɪlər/ *v.* 专门制作；定做

protocol /ˈproutəkɔːl/ *n.* 科学实验计划；医疗方案

nucleotide sequence 核苷酸序列

default /dɪˈfɔːlt/ *n.* 默认；系统设定值；预置值

pathology /pəˈθɑːlədʒi/ *n.* 病理学

precondition /ˌpriːkənˈdɪʃn/ *n.* 先决条件；前提

serotonin /ˌserəˈtounɪn/ *n.* 血清素，五羟色胺(神经递质，亦影响情绪等)

neurotransmitter /ˈnʊroutrænzmɪtər/ *n.* 神经递质

prone /proun/ *adj.* 易于遭受的；有做(坏事)倾向的

healthful /ˈhelθfl/ *adj.* 有益健康的

understanding of health should account for such preconditions. Moreover, health as absence of disease often depends upon personal and social values of what is health. Again, ambiguity enters into defining health given these values. For one person, health might be very different from that of another. The second notion of health does permit distinction between grades of health, in terms of quantifying it, and does not depend upon personal or social values. Proponents of this notion, such as Boorse, define health in terms of normal functioning, where the normal reflects a statistical norm with respect to species design. For example, a person with low levels of serotonin who is not clinically symptomatic in terms of depression is not as healthful as a person with statistically normal neurotransmitter levels. Criticisms of the second notion revolve around its lack of incorporating the social dimension of health and jettison the notion altogether opting for the notion of well-being. Well-being is a normative notion that combines both a person's values, especially in terms of his or her life goals, and objective physiological states. Because normative notions contain a person's value system, they are often difficult to define and defend since values vary from person to person and culture to culture.

In short, philosophers of medicine continue to debate a range of accounts: In broad outline, the most vigorous disagreement centers on whether more objective, biologically-based, and generalizable accounts are preferable to those that incorporate social and experiential perspectives. It is clear that none satisfy all of the desiderata of a complete and robust philosophical account that also can be useful for practitioners; although some would dispute whether the latter should be a requirement, many believe that philosophy of medicine should be responsive to and helpful for actual clinical practices.

New Expressions	
quantify /'kwɑːntɪfaɪ/ v. 以数量表述；量化	generalizable /'dʒenərəlaɪzəbl/ adj. 可概括的；可归纳的
symptomatic /ˌsɪmptə'mætɪk/ adj. 作为症状的；（有）症状的；作为征候的	preferable /'prefrəbl/ adj. 较适合的；更可取的
revolve /rɪ'vɑːlv/ v. 旋转；环绕；转动	desideratum /dɪˌzɪdə'rɑːtəm/ n. 需要的东西（pl. desiderata）
jettison /'dʒetɪsn/ v. 放弃；拒绝接受（想法、信念、计划等）	robust /roʊ'bʌst/ adj. 坚定的；信心十足的
opt /ɑːpt/ v. 选择；挑选	dispute /dɪ'spjuːt/ v. 对……提出质询；对……表示异议（或怀疑）
normative /'nɔːrmətɪv/ adj. 规范的；标准的	responsive /rɪ'spɑːnsɪv/ adj. 反应敏捷的；反应积极的
defend /dɪ'fend/ v. 辩解；辩白	
vigorous /'vɪɡərəs/ adj. 充满活力的；果断的；精力充沛的	

1. **lay persons:** 非专业人员，门外汉。Lay persons refer to persons who do not have expert knowledge of a particular subject.

2. **Tristram Engelhardt:** 崔斯特瑞姆·恩格尔哈特，1941—2018；美国哲学家，专攻医学史和医学哲学，主编丛书"哲学与医学"。他提出的疾病和健康等医学概念体现了生物伦理学和医学哲学的相互依赖。Engelhardt was one of the intellectual founders of the fields of bioethics and the philosophy of medicine, whose seminal work continues to frame debates about health care policy and medical practice.

3. **Christopher Boorse:** 克里斯托弗·波尔斯，1946 年至今；生物统计学理论（Bio-Statistical Theory，BST）的提出者。他认为，疾病是一种正常功能能力损伤的内部状态，没有能力以最低标准的效率实现所有典型的生理功能；而健康是简单的没有疾病，是各项参考类达到了统计上的正常函数，是生物统计研究的理论基础。在这一理论下，健康和疾病是经验的、客观的和无价值的概念。The liability for a naturalist definition of health and for a value-free distinction between the normal and the pathological is at the core of discussions on health and disease in philosophy of medicine. Boorse argues for BST which aims at solving these difficulties by articulating a statistical concept of normality and a non-normative concept of biological function.

Post-reading Activities

I **Language Building-up**

Task 1 **Extensive Vocabulary Enlargement**

Directions: *The following words are taken from the text. Please follow the three-step learning in this part and build up your own Extensive Vocabulary Chart.*

Step 1. Read through the words and underline them in the text. Circle the ones that are particularly new to you. Look up the words in the dictionary and put the equivalent Chinese translation in the chart on the next page.

Step 2. While you go back to the text, please feel free to put any other words into the blanks provided in the extra lines in the chart.

Extensive Vocabulary Chart				
maintain	asymptomatic	notoriously	variation	epistemologically
undesirable	critical	contentious	proponent	palpable
microorganism	champion	concrete	ambiguity	evolutionary
manifest	mutation	genomic	serotonin	generalizable

Step 3. Please group the above words based on their parts of speech and meanings.

Nouns	
Verbs	
Adjectives	
Adverbs and Prepositions	
Medical Terminology	
Terminology in Other Fields	

Directions: *The following 10 words are chosen from the text. They will form the intensive vocabulary in this unit. For intensive vocabulary, you are supposed to be able to explain them in English and use them in sentence and discourse constructions.*

Step 1. Please read through the words and be familiar with their Chinese and English definitions. Recall where and how they are used in the text.

No.	Word	Translation	Definition	Status
			Intensive Vocabulary Chart	
1	enjoin	命令；责令；嘱咐	*v.* to order or strongly advise sb. to do sth.; to say that a particular action or quality is necessary	☆☆☆☆☆
2	deviation	背离；偏离；违背	*n.* the act of moving away from what is normal or acceptable; a difference from what is expected or acceptable	☆☆☆☆☆
3	prone	易于遭受的；有做（坏事）的倾向的	*adj.* likely to suffer from sth. or to do sth. bad	☆☆☆☆☆
4	revolve	旋转；环绕；转动	*v.* to go in a circle around a central point	☆☆☆☆☆
5	jettison	（为减轻重量而从行驶的飞机或船上）扔弃，丢弃，投弃	*v.* to throw sth. out of a moving plane or ship to make it lighter	☆☆☆☆☆
6	defend	辩解；辩白	*v.* to say or write sth. in support of sb./sth. that has been criticized	☆☆☆☆☆
7	vigorous	充满活力的；果断的；精力充沛的	*adj.* very active, determined, or full of energy	☆☆☆☆☆
8	robust	坚定的；信心十足的	*adj.* strong and full of determination; showing that you are sure about what you are doing or saying	☆☆☆☆☆
9	dispute	对……提出质询；对……表示异议（或怀疑）	*v.* to question whether sth. is true and valid	☆☆☆☆☆
10	responsive	反应敏捷的；反应积极的	*adj.* reacting quickly and in a positive way	☆☆☆☆☆

Step 2. Please tick the status for each word based on your own situation. If one word is very new or difficult for you, please tick five stars. Likewise, if one word is comparatively easy for you and you don't have to spend too much time on reading and learning it, then tick one star. The number of stars represents the difficulty of commanding a word in your eyes.

Step 3. Please complete the following 10 sentences by choosing appropriate words from the Intensive Vocabulary Chart. Please change the forms of the words where necessary.

1. The earth _____ on its axis.
   地球环绕自身的轴心转动。

2. It is an unbearable act to _____ fuel into the sea.
   在大海中投弃燃料是不可容忍的行为。

3. Politicians are skilled at _____ themselves against their critics.
   从政者都善于为自己辩解，反驳别人的批评。

4. It is _____ whether the law applies in this case.
   有人对这项法律是否适用于这个案例提出质疑。

5. He _____ obedience on the soldiers.
   他命令士兵服从。

6. This is a(n) _____ campaign against tax fraud.
   这是一项坚决打击骗税的运动。

7. A flu virus that is not _____ to treatment makes people fearful.
   治疗无效的流感病毒让人害怕。

8. Any _____ from the party's faith is seen as betrayal.
   任何对党的信仰的偏离都被视作背叛。

9. It was a typically _____ performance by the Foreign Secretary.
   这是外交大臣典型的有信心的表现。

10. Working without a break makes you more _____ to error.
    连续不停歇地工作使你更容易出错。

Task 3　Expressions and Sentences

Directions: *The following sentences are taken from the text. In each sentence, there are one or two phrases being underlined. Please refer to the dictionary and write down the explanation of the phrases in the line entitled "Meaning Exploration". After that, please choose one phrase and make a sentence with it. Write the sentence in the line entitled "Sentence Making".*

Sentence 1

Original Sentence	Thus the dividing line between disease and health is notoriously vague, due in part to the wide range of variations present in the human population and to debates over whether many concepts of disease are socially constructed.
Meaning Exploration	*due to*: *in part*:
Sentence Making	

Sentence 2

Original Sentence	Critics who object to this notion, however, cite the ambiguity of the term "norm" in terms of a reference class.
Meaning Exploration	*object to*:
Sentence Making	

Sentence 3

Original Sentence	The genetic notion claims that disease is the mutation in or absence of a gene.
Meaning Exploration	*absence of*:
Sentence Making	

Sentence 4

Original Sentence	An adequate understanding of health should account for such preconditions.
Meaning Exploration	*account for*:
Sentence Making	

Sentence 5

Original Sentence	Moreover, health as absence of disease often <u>depends upon</u> personal and social values of what is health.
Meaning Exploration	*depend upon:*
Sentence Making	

II Critical Reading and Thinking

Task 1   Overview and Comprehension

Directions: *In the text, the author has presented several different notions of disease and health respectively. Please summarize the notions in the following chart based on what you have read from the text.*

Concepts	Different Notions
Disease	
Health	

Task 2   Reflection and Discussion

Directions: *After reading, please reflect on the theme of the text. Work in groups and share your opinions on the following questions with other group members.*

1. What's the purpose of exploring the distinction between health and disease? Is it important? Why or why not?

2. Which notion of disease would you agree with or disagree with? Please choose one and share your thoughts on it.

3. Which notion of health would you agree with or disagree with? Please choose one and share your thoughts on it.

4. If you were a philosopher of medicine, how would you like to draw the dividing line between disease and health?

Part 3 Extended Reading

*Being Mortal*①1

…

He was alive just four more days, as it turned out. When I arrived at his bedside, I found him **alert** and unhappy about **awaking** in the hospital. No one listens to him, he said. He'd awoken in severe pain but the medical staff wouldn't give him enough **medication** to stop it, fearing he might lose consciousness again. I asked the nurse to give him the full dose he took at home. She had to get permission from the doctor **on call**, and still he approved only half.

Finally, at 3:00 a.m., my father had had enough. He began shouting. He demanded that they take out his **IVs**[2] and let him go home. "Why are you doing nothing?" he yelled. "Why are you letting me suffer?" He'd become **incoherent** with pain. He called the Cleveland Clinic—two hundred miles away—on his cell phone and told a confused doctor on duty to "Do something." His night nurse finally got permission for a **slug** of an intravenous **narcotic**, but he refused it. "It doesn't work," he said. Finally, at 5:00 a.m., we **persuaded** him to take the injection, and the pain began to **subside**. He became calm. But he still wanted to go home. In a hospital built to ensure survival at all costs and unclear how to do otherwise, he understood his choices would never be his own.

New Expressions	
alert /ə'lɜːrt/ *adj.* 警觉的；警惕的；戒备的	**slug** /slʌg/ *n.* 少量
awake /ə'weɪk/ *v.* （使）醒来	**narcotic** /nɑːr'kɑːtɪk/ *n.* 镇静剂；麻醉药；催眠药
medication /ˌmedɪ'keɪʃn/ *n.* 药；药物	**persuade** /pər'sweɪd/ *v.* 劝说；说服
on call （医生、警察等）随叫随到（尤其是在紧急情况下）	**subside** /səb'saɪd/ *v.* 趋于平静；平息；减弱；消退
incoherent /ˌɪnkoʊ'hɪrənt/ *adj.* 口齿不清的；语无伦次的	

---

① The text is adapted from the following source: Gawande, A. 2014. *Being Mortal: Medicine and What Matters in the End*. New York: Metropolitan Books.

We arranged for the medical staff to give him his morning dose of medication, stop his oxygen and his **antibiotics** for his pneumonia, and let us take him. By **midmorning**, he was back in his bed.

"I do not want suffering," he repeated when he had me alone. "Whatever happens, will you promise me you won't let me suffer?"

"Yes," I said.

That was harder to achieve than it would seem. Just **urinating**, for instance, proved a problem. His **paralysis** had advanced from just the week before, and one sign was that he became unable to pee. He could still feel when his **bladder** became full but could make nothing come out. I helped him to the bathroom and **swiveled** him onto the seat. Then I waited while he sat there. Half an hour passed. "It'll come," he insisted. He tried not to think about it. He pointed out the toilet seat from Lowe's he'd had **installed** a couple months before. It was **electric**, he said. He loved it. It could wash his bottom with a **burst** of water and dry it. No one had to wipe him. He could take care of himself.

"Have you tried it?" he asked.

"That would be no," I said.

"You ought to," he said, smiling.

But still nothing came out. Then the bladder **spasms** began. He **groaned** when they came over him. "You're going to have to **catheterize** me," he said. The **hospice**[3] nurse, expecting this moment would come, had brought the supplies and trained my mother. But I'd done it a hundred times for my own patients. So I pulled my father up from the seat, got him back to bed, and set about doing it for him, his eyes **squeezed** shut the entire time. It's not something a person ever thinks he/she will come to. But I got the

New Expressions	
antibiotic /ˌæntibaɪˈɑːtɪk/ n. 抗菌素；抗生素	electric /ɪˈlektrɪk/ adj. 电的；用电的；电动的；发电的
midmorning /ˌmɪdˈmɔːrnɪŋ/ n. 早晨；上午	burst /bɜːrst/ n. 突发；猝发；迸发；爆破
urinate /ˈjʊrəneɪt/ v. 排尿；小便	spasm /ˈspæzəm/ n. 痉挛；抽搐
paralysis /pəˈræləsɪs/ n. 麻痹；瘫痪	groan /ɡroʊn/ v. 呻吟；叹息；哼哼
bladder /ˈblædər/ n. 膀胱	catheterize /ˈkæθətəˌraɪz/ v. 插入导管；将导管插入
swivel /ˈswɪvl/ v.（使）旋转；转动	squeeze /skwiːz/ v. 挤压；捏
install /ɪnˈstɔːl/ v. 安装；设置	

catheter in, and the urine flooded out. The relief was oceanic.

His greatest struggle remained the pain from his tumor—not because it was difficult to control but because it was difficult to agree on how much to control it. By the third day, he'd become unarousable again for long periods. The question became whether to keep giving him his regular dose of liquid morphine, which could be put under his tongue where it would absorb into his bloodstream through his mucous membranes. My sister and I thought we should, fearing that he might wake up in pain. My mother thought we shouldn't, fearing the opposite.

"Maybe if he had a little pain, he'd wake up," she said, her eyes welling. "He still has so much he can do."

Even in his last couple of days, she was not wrong. When he was permitted to rise above the demands of his body, he took the opportunity for small pleasures greedily. He could still enjoy certain foods and ate surprisingly well, asking for chapatis, rice, curried string beans, potatoes, yellow split-pea dahl, black-eyed-pea chutney, and *shira*[4], a sweet dish from his youth. He talked to his grandchildren by phone. He sorted photos. He gave instructions about unfinished projects. He had but the tiniest fragments of life left that he could grab, and we were agonizing over them. Could we get him another one?

Nonetheless, I remembered my pledge to him and gave him his morphine every two hours, as planned. My mother anxiously accepted it. For long hours, he lay quiet and stock-still, except for the rattle of his breathing. He'd have a sharp intake of breath—it sounded like a snore that would shut off suddenly, as if a lid had come down—

New Expressions	
catheter /ˈkæθɪtər/ n. 导管（如导尿管）	chutney /ˈtʃʌtni/ n. 酸辣酱
urine /ˈjurən/ n. 尿；小便	sort /sɔːrt/ v. 整理；把……分类
oceanic /ˌoʊʃiˈænɪk/ adj. 海洋的；大海的；与海洋有关的	fragment /ˈfrægmənt/ n. 碎片；片段
	agonize /ˈægənaɪz/ v. 苦苦思索；焦虑不已
unarousable /ˌʌnəˈraʊzəbl/ adj. 不可被唤醒的	pledge /pledʒ/ n. 保证；诺言；誓约
morphine /ˈmɔːrfiːn/ n. 吗啡	stock-still /ˌstɑːk ˈstɪl/ adj. 静止的；一动不动的
absorb /əbˈsɔːrb/ v. 吸收（液体、气体）	rattle /ˈrætl/ n. 一连串短促尖厉的撞击声；咔嗒声
mucous membrane 黏膜	
greedily /ˈgriːdɪli/ adv. 贪心地；贪婪地	snore /snɔːr/ n. 打呼噜（声）；打鼾（声）
chapati /tʃəˈpɑːti/ n.（印度）薄煎饼	shut off 停止
dahl /dɑːl/ n. 印度扁豆（菜肴）	lid /lɪd/ n.（容器的）盖，盖子

followed a second later by a long **exhalation**. The air rushing past the **mucoid** fluid in his windpipe sounded like someone shaking **pebbles** in a hollow tube in his chest. Then there'd be silence for what seemed like forever before the cycle would start up again.

…

Later, we wheeled him to the dinner table. He had some mangoes, papayas, yogurt, and his medications. He was silent, breathing normally again, thinking.

"What are you thinking?" I asked.

"I'm thinking how to not **prolong** the process of dying. This—this food prolongs the process."

My mom didn't like hearing this.

"We're happy taking care of you, Ram," she said. "We love you."

He shook his head.

"It's hard, isn't it?" my sister said.

"Yes. It's hard."

"If you could sleep through it, is that what you'd prefer?" I asked.

"Yes."

"You don't want to be awake, aware of us, with us like this?" my mother asked.

He didn't say anything for a moment. We waited.

"I don't want to experience this," he said.

The suffering my father experienced in his final day was not exactly physical. The medicine did a good job of preventing pain. When he surfaced **periodically**, at the **tide** of consciousness, he would smile at our voices. But then he'd be fully **ashore** and realize

New Expressions	
exhalation /ˌeksʃəˈleɪʃn/ *n.* 呼出；呼气；蒸发；发散物	**periodically** /ˌpɪriˈɑːdɪkli/ *adv.* 周期性地；定期地；间发性地
mucoid /ˈmjuˌkɔɪd/ *adj.* 类黏蛋白的；似黏液的；黏液状的	**tide** /taɪd/ *n.* 高涨的情绪；潮；潮汐；潮水
pebble /ˈpebl/ *n.* 鹅卵石；砾石	**ashore** /əˈʃɔːr/ *adv.* 向（或在）岸上；向（或在）陆地
prolong /prəˈlɔːŋ/ *v.* 延长	

that it was not over. He'd realize that all the anxieties of enduring that he'd hoped would be gone were still there: The problems with his body, yes, but more difficult for him the problems with his mind—the confusion, the worries about his unfinished work, about mom, about how he'd be remembered. He was at peace in sleep, not in wakefulness. And what he wanted for the final lines of his story, now that nature was pressing its limits, was peacefulness.

During his final **bout** of wakefulness, he asked for the grandchildren. They were not there, so I showed him pictures on my iPad. His eyes went wide, and his smile was huge. He looked at every picture in detail.

Then he **descended** back **into** unconsciousness. His breathing stopped for twenty or thirty seconds at a time. I'd be sure it was over, only to find that his breathing would start again. It went on this way for hours.

Finally, around ten after six in the afternoon, while my mother and sister were talking and I was reading a book, I noticed that he'd stopped breathing for longer than before.

"I think he's stopped," I said.

We went to him. My mother took his hand. And we listened, each of us silent.

No more breaths came.

New Expressions	
bout /baʊt/ *n.* 一阵；一场；（尤指坏事的）一通，一次	**descend** /dɪˈsend/ *v.* 下来；下去；下降 **descend into** 逐渐陷入

Notes

1. *Being Mortal*:《最好的告别》。本书是哈佛医学院教授、医生阿图·葛文德（Atul Gawande）于 2014 年出版的非虚构书籍，讲述了衰老与死亡的故事，以及如何有尊严地迎接死亡。*Being Mortal* is a meditation on how people can better live with age-related frailty, serious illness, and approaching death. Gawande calls for a change in the way that medical professionals treat patients approaching their ends. He recommends that instead of focusing on survival, practitioners should work to improve their quality of life and enable their well-being.

2. IVs: 静脉注射，其全称为 intravenous injections。静脉注射是一种医疗方法，即把血液、药液、营养液等液体物质直接注射到静脉中。

3. hospice: 临终关怀。临终关怀是指为疾病终末期或老年患者在临终前提供身体、心理、精神等方面的照料和人文关怀等服务，控制痛苦和不适症状，提高生命质量，帮助患者舒适、安详、有尊严地离世。Hospice care is a type of health care that focuses on the palliation of a terminally ill patient's pain and symptoms and attending to their emotional and spiritual needs at the end of life. Hospice care prioritizes comfort and quality of life by reducing pain and suffering. Hospice care provides an alternative to therapies focused on life-prolonging measures that may be arduous, likely to cause more symptoms, or are not aligned with a person's goals.

4. *shira*: 也称 *sheera* 或 *suji halwa*，是一种传统印度甜品，由粗面粉、酥油、糖、腰果和葡萄干制成。*Shira* is a type of traditional dessert in India.

Post-reading Activities

I **Speaking Practice: Role play**

Directions: *Please work in pairs. Imagine one of you is the author of the text, and the other is the father who is tired of the suffering he experienced to prolong life in his final days. Please design a conversation between the author and his father during which the author asks about his father's needs and preferences for medical treatment in his last few days. Be sure to present the complicated feelings the author may have while discussing end-of-life matters with his own father. Please take turns to be the author and the father.*

II **Reflective Writing Practice: Short Essay**

Directions: *In his book* Being Mortal, *Gawande said: "When you are young and healthy, you believe you will live forever. But when you see the future ahead of you as finite and uncertain—your focus shifts to everyday pleasures and the people closest to you." Please think about the biological, social, and psychological status a person might experience at the end of his or her life course and write a reflective essay entitled "What Matters in the End". The word limit is suggested to be 150–200 words.*

Unit 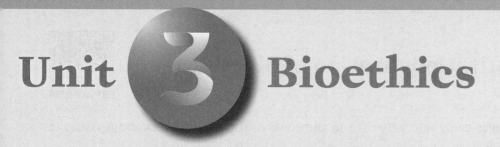 Bioethics

> *To live an ethical life is not self-sacrifice, but self-fulfillment.*
> *—Peter Singer*

The First Use of Ether in Dental Surgery, by Ernest Board, 1846

Part 1 Academic Horizon

Institutionalization of Bioethics[①]

Bioethics came into existence in the context of public debates about issues in (bio)medical science. The institutionalization of bioethics is mostly a consequence of the increasing need of **parliaments**, governments and churches to obtain advice on ethical questions in the light of developments in medical science and biotechnology. Numerous ethics committees have been formed to fulfill this need. The functions of these institutions vary. Some committees were established merely to advise on concrete, well-defined questions; others are permanent advisory boards concerned with a whole range of societally relevant questions in the domain of the biosciences or other new technologies. While varied in assignment, they are also varied in size and **composition**. As a rule, these committees are interdisciplinary (with physicians, jurists, philosophers and **theologians**) and they usually consist not only of academics, but of representatives of relevant parties in society as well (churches, disability rights advocates, etc.).

Besides ethical advisory boards **affiliated** with political institutions, committees have also been formed to advise researchers and hospitals. These so-called "ethics committee" at medical faculties are **geared** towards **verifying** that the protection of medical test subjects with regard to risks and informed consent is guaranteed. The title "ethics committee" for these bodies is somewhat misleading, since their intention is not to carry out ethical **reflection** on the research project at issue, but merely to certify that

New Expressions	
institutionalization /ˌɪnstɪˌtuːʃənələˈzeɪʃn/ *n.* 制度化	**theologian** /ˌθiːəˈləʊdʒn/ *n.* 神学家
bioethics /ˌbaɪəʊˈeθɪks/ *n.* 生物伦理学，生命伦理学（影响医学和生物学研究的道德准则）	**affiliate** /əˈfɪlɪeɪt/ *v.* 与……有关；为……工作
	gear /ɡɪr/ *v.* 使与……相适应；使适合于
parliament /ˈpɑːrləmənt/ *n.* 议会；国会	**verify** /ˈverɪfaɪ/ *v.* 核实；查对；核准
composition /ˌkɑːmpəˈzɪʃn/ *n.* 成分；构成；组合方式	**reflection** /rɪˈflekʃn/ *n.* 沉思；深思；审慎的思考

① The text is adapted from the following source: Düwell, M. 2012. *Bioethics: Methods, Theories, Domains*. Oxfordshire: Routledge.

 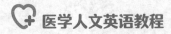 医学人文英语教程

the relevant codes of conduct are observed. These committees are standardly composed of physicians, **complemented** by a (theological or philosophical) ethicist and a jurist.

In recent years, clinical ethics committees and institutionalized forms of ethics advisory boards in hospitals have also been created, to which doctors, nurses and patients can turn in case of conflicts and difficult decisions in treatment and nursing. The task of these advisory services is geared towards individual cases, and is typically not very well defined. Mainly, the point is to create a space within the clinical **praxis** in which conflict situations can be dealt with **transparently** with regard to both argumentation and procedure. It may be that, as a rule, these committees are forums that are partially about conflict **moderation** and the protection of decision-makers. But in any case they are places that should make it possible for difficult practical situations to be dealt with in morally responsible ways.

With these three types of committees, the contexts in which bioethics emerged have already been laid out. From the start, the objective of bioethics was to advise and reflect on complex decisions in politics, research and clinical practice. In the domain of medicine, more and more situations arose in which the traditional ethical guidelines of the discipline were not helpful, for which moral intuitions were not prepared, and in which there were no or insufficient legal arrangements to guide a decision-making process. In these contexts, the expression "bioethics" **signaled** first and foremost a need for reflection on the moral and legal standards regulating medical practice, as well as a need for guidance on the part of decision-makers. It is still undefined, however, in what ways this specific form of advice and reflection differs from other kinds of conflict moderation. And it is even less clear how the advisory task of these boards relates to what has been established as "bioethics" in academic **spheres**.

In addition, this advisory task turns out to differ greatly between the forms of institutionalization discussed. A clinical ethics committee is confronted with particular cases. As a rule, these particular cases are settled against a backdrop of legal regulations, established practices and widely shared moral **convictions**. However, the great need

New Expressions	
complement /'kɑːmplɪmənt/ v. 补充；补足；使完美；使更具吸引力	**moderation** /ˌmɑːdə'reɪʃn/ n. 适度；适中；合理；缓和
praxis /'præksɪs/ n. 做事方法；实践；实际应用	**signal** /'sɪɡnəl/ v. 标志；表明；预示
	sphere /sfɪr/ n. 范围；领域；阶层；界
transparently /træns'pærəntli/ adv. 易懂地；明晰地	**conviction** /kən'vɪkʃn/ n. 坚定的看法（或信念）

for ethical advice indicates that ever more practices are becoming problematic, and ever fewer moral convictions can be taken for granted as shared. Nonetheless, no comprehensive ethical theories are called upon when such conflict situations are being dealt with in medical practice. Rather, those involved tend to fall back on medical knowledge, somewhat familiar standards of medical and nursing practice and moral principles that are considered to be unproblematic. Incidentally, the customs of medical practice are based only in part on the question whether those acts could meet with general approval in the public sphere. The medical profession has simply been successful in **asserting** certain standards of medical practice within its strongly hierarchically organized and legally **regulated** domain. In any case, factual **observance** of a given standard and its moral acceptance are two different things for ethical advice is thus also an **indicator** for the necessity to think about established forms of practice.

New Expressions
assert /əˈsɜːrt/ v. 明确肯定；断言   遵守，奉行
regulate /ˈreɡjʊleɪt/ v. 管理；调节   **indicator** /ˈɪndɪkeɪtər/ n. 指示信号；标志
observance /əbˈzɜːrvəns/ n.（对法律、习俗的）

Post-reading Activities

I Speaking Practice: Group Discussion

Directions: *Please discuss the following questions in small groups. After your discussion, please share your opinions with the whole class.*

1. What causes the institutionalization of bioethics?
2. What is known about the composition of ethics committees?
3. How many different types of ethics committees are mentioned in the text? What are they?
4. What is the objective of bioethics?

II Speaking Practice: Oral Presentation

Directions: *From the text, it is known that there are ethics committees created both at medical faculties and in hospitals. What are the differences and similarities between them? Please compare the two and write down what you find in the following chart. After that, please present your comparison and reflection on the practices of these committees. You are welcome to give criticism and suggestions on improving the practices of ethics committees.*

	Ethics Committees at Medical Faculties	Ethics Committees in Hospitals
Similarities		
Differences		
Reflections on Their Practices		

Part 2 Thematic Reading

Ethical Issues in Assisted Reproductive Medicine[①]

Louise Brown, the First Test Tube Baby

Test tube **conception** is the popular name for **in vitro fertilization (IVF)**. It involves fertilization outside the **womb**, in a **Petri dish**[1]. Lesley Brown, the mother of the first child **conceived** in vitro, had damaged **fallopian tubes** from **ectopic** pregnancies. For her IVF, scientists removed one of her eggs and placed it in a Petri dish, where they mixed her husband John's **sperm** to form an **embryo**. With the embryo returned to her **uterus**, Lesley then carried it to normal **gestation**.

Two decades of research by **Robert Edwards**[2], a **physiologist** at Cambridge University, **preceded** the first IVF birth. Over the two decades, the researcher and his team attempted IVF many times. Their 102nd attempt resulted in Louise Brown. In 1977, **Dr. Steptoe**[3] told Lesley she was pregnant. Before this, some women had had eggs successfully **fertilized** in vitro, but all had lost the embryo. Lesley made it to five months, and her **amniocentesis** showed a normal pregnancy. She spent the last month of her

New Expressions	
conception /kən'sepʃn/ *n.* 怀孕；受孕	**embryo** /'embriou/ *n.* 胚；胚胎
in vitro 在生物体外进行；在科学仪器中进行	**uterus** /'juːtərəs/ *n.* 子宫
fertilization /ˌfɜːrtələ'zeɪʃn/ *n.* 受精	**gestation** /dʒe'steɪʃn/ *n.* 妊娠（期）；怀孕（期）
IVF /ˌaɪviː'ef/ *n.* 体外受精；试管受精	**physiologist** /ˌfɪzi'ɑːlədʒɪst/ *n.* 生理学家
womb /wuːm/ *n.* 子宫	**precede** /prɪ'siːd/ *v.* 在……之前发生（或出现）；先于
conceive /kən'siːv/ *v.* 怀孕；怀胎	**fertilize** /'fɜːrtəlaɪz/ *v.* 使受孕
fallopian tube 输卵管	**amniocentesis** /ˌæmniousen'tiːsɪs/ *n.* 羊膜穿刺术
ectopic /ek'tɑːpɪk/ *adj.* （妊娠）异位的，子宫外的	
sperm /spɜːrm/ *n.* 精子	

---

① The text is adapted from the following source: Pence, G. E. 2017. *Medical Ethics: Accounts of Ground-breaking Cases.* New York: McGraw-Hill Education.

 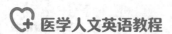

pregnancy at Oldham Hospital **under siege** by the media. Steptoe delivered the baby, a girl, by **cesarean** section on July 25, 1978. Between 1978, which saw the world's first test tube baby, and now, assisted reproduction raised many ethical issues.

Payment for Assisted Reproduction: Egg Donors

Originally, young volunteers supplied eggs for older women, but **altruism** didn't meet the demand. Paying for eggs is **euphemistically** called "egg donation", and in America in 2016, clinics in New York City paid egg donors $8,000 per cycle.

Egg **retrieval** is more complicated than obtaining sperm. A woman takes drugs daily for a month or more to induce **superovulation**, after which eggs are **aspirated** as previously explained. Some people claim that the drugs increase risk of some cancers over the life of the woman, but no long-term data support this claim.

In 1999, a famous ad ran in newspapers at Princeton and Yale Universities, stating that an **anonymous** couple would pay $50,000 for the eggs of a "woman over six feet tall and with SAT[4] scores over 1,450". Payment also runs high for donors of Jewish or Asian background, because they donate less frequently. Critics rarely complained when clinics paid males to donate sperm, even though genetically sperm and eggs are both **gametes** and contain the same amount of genetic information. Critics mainly **condemn** payment of women for eggs.

Payment for Assisted Reproduction: Adoption

Because roughly 1 out of 11 couples in North America is **infertile** after a year of trying to conceive, and IVF works for only 20 couples out of 100, infertile couples create high demand for healthy, adoptable babies. Because most adopting couples in North America are "white" and want a "white" child, demand for such babies has **skyrocketed**.

New Expressions	
under siege 受围攻；遭受严厉批评；承受巨大压力	**anonymous** /ə'nɑːnɪməs/ *adj.* 不知姓名的；名字不公开的
cesarean /sɪ'zerɪən/ *n.* 剖腹产	**gamete** /'gæmiːt/ *n.* 配子
altruism /'æltrʊɪzəm/ *n.* 利他主义	**condemn** /kən'dem/ *v.* （通常因道义而）谴责，指责
euphemistically /ˌjuːfə'mɪstɪkli/ *adv.* 委婉地	
retrieval /rɪ'triːvl/ *n.* 取回；索回	**adoption** /ə'dɑːpʃn/ *n.* 收养；领养
superovulation /ˌsuːpərˌɑvjə'leɪʃn/ *n.* 超数排卵	**infertile** /ɪn'fɜːrtl/ *adj.* 不育的；不结果实的
aspirate /'æspəreɪt/ *v.* （用吸引机）抽吸（体腔中的液体）	**skyrocket** /'skaɪrɑːkɪt/ *v.* 飞涨；猛涨

As a result, the average couple in 2015 seeking to adopt a baby paid private agencies $28,000.

Like transfer of eggs or organs, agencies do not technically sell babies, which is illegal. But a new industry has **sprung up** that connects couples to pregnant women who might put their babies up for adoption. According to one investigative journalist, "That has left only the thinnest line between buying a child and buying adoption services that lead to a child." The doubling of licensed child placement has increased adoptions in North America in the last few years to nearly 2,000.

Although "black" critics have recently **decried** the lesser payments that seem to **demean** "black" babies, virtually no one has condemned payment itself. No one has criticized "pregnancy counseling centers" that encourage pregnant girls to give up their babies for adoption, while charging $30,000 to couples who adopt those babies.

Gender Selection

Because X **chromosomes** weigh more than Y chromosomes, Microsort, a modified flow **cytometer,** can separate heavier from lighter sperm, producing accurate results 90 percent of the time. Although intended for **pre-implantation** genetic **diagnosis**, Microsort may be used to select male babies.

Gender selection is an issue in many countries, where parents saw females as less desirable than males. Using **sonograms**, many families **aborted** female **fetuses** to try again for a male child. Sex selection is sexist and leads to **imbalances** of the sexes in the population. It should be banned.

Unnatural

In 1978, the year of Louise Brown's birth, **the Vatican**[5] condemned IVF and has not changed its position since. Its instructions of 1987 **equated** IVF with "domination" and

New Expressions	
spring /sprɪŋ/ v. 突然出现	**diagnosis** /ˌdaɪəɡ'noʊsɪs/ n. 诊断；（问题原因的）判断
spring up 迅速出现；突然兴起	
decry /dɪ'kraɪ/ v.（公开）谴责；（强烈）批评	**sonogram** /'sɑːnəˌɡræm/ n. 声波图
demean /dɪ'miːn/ v. 贬低；贬损；使失尊严	**abort** /ə'bɔːrt/ v. 使流产
chromosome /'krəʊməsəʊm/ n. 染色体	**fetus** /'fiːtəs/ n. 胎儿
cytometer /saɪ'tɑːmɪtər/ n. 血细胞计数器	**imbalance** /ɪm'bæləns/ n. 失衡；不平衡；不公平
pre-implantation /prɪˌɪmplæn'teɪʃn/ n. 胚胎植前	**equate** /i'kweɪt/ v. 同等看待；使等同

"**manipulation** of nature". In 2008, in "Dignity of the Person", it emphasized that children should be created only through sexual intercourse of a married couple. The document bans IVF, freezing embryos, and **screening** them genetically.

Paul Ramsey, a socially conservative Protestant theologian at Princeton University, in 1970 equated IVF with genetic manipulation, predicting societal horrors to such a practice. He implied that if physicians could find a tiny egg and fertilize it, why couldn't they **alter** its genes? He predicted that if they could, they would, and he held that if they did, it would be **sinful**.

When Lesley Brown was several months pregnant, at the invitation of Sargent Shriver, Robert Edwards attended a **symposium** on the ethics of IVF at Washington's Kennedy Institute for Bioethics. While **senators**, national columnists, and other scientists listened, Ramsey condemned IVF. Ramsey condemned IVF not based on its possible harmful consequences to the child, to the parents, or to society, but rather, and in a view that resurfaced 20 years later, from the idea of wronging the embryo-person. IVF is wrong in itself, Ramsey held, because it is "**unconsented-to** experimentation" on a person, the embryo.

Besides the above mentioned issues, people also criticized that reproductive medicine has created physical and psychological harm to babies born in new ways and has **deprived** their rights of knowing their biological parents. Should reproductive medicine be promoted and **commercialized**? It is indeed time to regulate the Fertility Clinics.

New Expressions	
manipulation /mə.nɪpju'leɪʃn/ *n.*（暗中）控制，操纵；影响	**senator** /'senətər/ *n.* 参议员
screen /skriːn/ *v.* 筛查；检查	**unconsented-to** /ˌʌnkən'sentɪd tuː/ *adj.* 未经许可的
alter /'ɔːltər/ *v.*（使）改变，更改，改动	**deprive** /dɪ'praɪv/ *v.* 剥夺；使丧失；使不能享有
sinful /'sɪnfl/ *adj.* 不道德的；邪恶的	
symposium /sɪm'pəʊziəm/ *n.* 专题讨论会；研讨会；小型讨论会	**commercialize** /kə'mɜːrʃəlaɪz/ *v.*（尤指不择手段地）利用……牟利；商业化

1. **Petri dish:** 皮氏培养皿。皮氏培养皿是一种带盖子的玻璃制品，生物学家可用其培养细胞、细菌、真菌和微型苔藓等，由德国细菌学家朱利斯·理查德·佩特里发明，因此而得名。A Petri dish is a shallow transparent lidded dish that biologists use to hold growth media in which cells can be cultured, originally, cells of bacteria, fungi, and small mosses. The container is named after its inventor, German bacteriologist Julius Richard Petri.

2. **Robert Edwards:** 罗伯特·爱德华兹，1925—2013；英国生理学家、剑桥大学教授，被誉为"试管婴儿之父"。In 2010, Edwards was awarded the Nobel Prize in Physiology or Medicine "for the development of in vitro fertilization".

3. **Dr. Steptoe:** 全名为 Patrick Christopher Steptoe（帕特里克·克里斯托弗·斯特普托），1913—1988；英国发明家、体外受精和试管婴儿技术的发明者。他曾与罗伯特·爱德华兹一起合作，发展了人体医学的体外受精技术，二者合作成就了人类历史上的第一个试管婴儿。Dr. Steptoe has collaborated with Robert Edward in the development of IVF. Their collaboration has enabled the birth of the first IVF child in human history.

4. **SAT:** 全称是 Scholastic Assessment Test。SAT 是由美国大学委员会主办的一种考试，其成绩是世界各国高中生申请美国大学入学资格及奖学金的重要参考。The SAT is a standardized test designed to measure basic critical reading, math and writing skills. The SAT offers colleges a detailed profile of student skills and strengths, informing strategic recruiting efforts and admission decisions.

5. **the Vatican:** 梵蒂冈（罗马教皇的驻地）。梵蒂冈是指在西方世界至高无上的罗马教廷、教皇权力。The Vatican is the center of the government of the Roman Catholic Church. It is also a metonym for the Holy See.

Post-reading Activities

I Language Building-up

Task 1 Extensive Vocabulary Enlargement

Directions: *The following words are taken from the text. Please follow the three-step learning in this part and build up your own Extensive Vocabulary Chart.*

Step 1. Read through the words and underline them in the text. Circle the ones that are particularly new to you. Look up the words in the dictionary and put the equivalent Chinese translation in the chart below.

Step 2. While you go back to the text, please feel free to put any other words into the blanks provided in the extra lines in the chart.

Extensive Vocabulary Chart				
conception	womb	uterus	gestation	physiologist
fertilize	amniocentesis	cesarean	altruism	superovulation
anonymous	gamete	chromosome	cytometer	sonogram
fetus	manipulation	screen	sinful	senator

Step 3. Please group the above words based on their parts of speech and meanings.

Nouns	
Verbs	

Adjectives	
Adverbs and Prepositions	
Medical Terminology	
Terminology in Other Fields	

Task 2　Intensive Vocabulary Enhancement

Directions: *The following 10 words are chosen from the text. They will form the intensive vocabulary in this unit. For intensive vocabulary, you are supposed to be able to explain them in English and use them in sentence and discourse constructions.*

Step 1.　Please read through the words and be familiar with their Chinese and English definitions. Recall where and how they are used in the text.

		Intensive Vocabulary Chart		
No.	Word	Translation	Definition	Status
1	conceive	怀孕；怀胎	*v.* to become pregnant	☆ ☆ ☆ ☆ ☆
2	condemn	（通常因道义而）谴责，指责	*v.* to express very strong disapproval of sb./sth., usually for moral reasons	☆ ☆ ☆ ☆ ☆
3	skyrocket	（价格等）飞涨，猛涨	*v.* (of prices, etc.) to rise quickly to a very high level	☆ ☆ ☆ ☆ ☆
4	decry	（公开）谴责；（强烈）批评	*v.* (formal) to strongly criticize sb./sth., especially publicly	☆ ☆ ☆ ☆ ☆
5	demean	贬低；贬损；使失尊严	*v.* to make people have less respect for sb./sth.	☆ ☆ ☆ ☆ ☆
6	equate	同等看待；使等同	*v.* to think that sth. is the same as sth. else or is as important	☆ ☆ ☆ ☆ ☆
7	alter	（使）改变,更改,改动	*v.* to become different; to make sb./sth. different	☆ ☆ ☆ ☆ ☆

Intensive Vocabulary Chart				
No.	Word	Translation	Definition	Status
8	consent	同意；准许；允许	*v.* (rather formal) to agree to sth. or give your permission for sth.	☆ ☆ ☆ ☆ ☆
9	deprive	剥夺；使丧失；使不能享有	*v.* to prevent sb. from having or doing sth., especially sth. important	☆ ☆ ☆ ☆ ☆
10	commercialize	（尤指不择手段地）利用……牟利；商业化	*v.* to use sth. to try to make a profit, especially in a way that other people do not approve of	☆ ☆ ☆ ☆ ☆

Step 2. Please tick the status for each word based on your own situation. If one word is very new or difficult for you, please tick five stars. Likewise, if one word is comparatively easy for you and you don't have to spend too much time on reading and learning it, then tick one star. The number of stars represents the difficulty of commanding a word in your eyes.

Step 3. Please complete the following 10 sentences by choosing appropriate words from the Intensive Vocabulary Chart. Please change the forms of the words where necessary.

1. Some parents _____ education with exam success.
   有些父母认为教育就是考试成绩优秀。

2. He had _____ so much I scarcely recognized him.
   他变得我几乎认不出来了。

3. They were imprisoned and _____ of their basic rights.
   他们遭到监禁并被剥夺了基本权利。

4. The fact that she could not _____ has almost driven her crazy.
   她不能怀孕这件事快把她逼疯了。

5. The measures were _____ as useless.
   这些措施受到指责，说是不起作用。

6. Their music has become very _____ in recent years.
   近几年，他们的音乐已经非常商业化了。

7. I don't like those images that _____ women.
   我不喜欢那些有损妇女尊严的图像。

8. The government issued a statement _____ the bribery.
   政府发表声明谴责这起行贿事件。

9. The price of sugar has suddenly _____ up.

糖价突然飞涨。

10. When she told them what she intended, they readily _____

她把打算告诉他们时，他们欣然同意。

Task 3　Expressions and Sentences

Directions: *The following sentences are taken from the text. In each sentence, there is one phrase being underlined. Please refer to the dictionary and write down the explanation of the phrase in the line entitled "Meaning Exploration". After that, please make a sentence with it. Write the sentence in the line entitled "Sentence Making".*

Sentence 1

Original Sentence	She spent the last month of her pregnancy at Oldham Hospital under siege by the media.
Meaning Exploration	under siege:
Sentence Making	

Sentence 2

Original Sentence	Originally, young volunteers supplied eggs for older women, but altruism didn't meet the demand.
Meaning Exploration	meet the demand:
Sentence Making	

Sentence 3

Original Sentence	Some people claim that the drugs increase risk of some cancers over the life of the woman, but no long-term data support this claim.
Meaning Exploration	increase risk of:
Sentence Making	

Sentence 4

Original Sentence	But a new industry has <u>sprung up</u> that connects couples to pregnant women who might put their babies up for adoption.
Meaning Exploration	*spring up*:
Sentence Making	

Sentence 5

Original Sentence	When Lesley Brown was several months pregnant, <u>at the invitation of</u> Sargent Shriver, Robert Edwards attended a symposium on the ethics of IVF at Washington's Kennedy Institute for Bioethics.
Meaning Exploration	*at the invitation of*:
Sentence Making	

II Critical Reading and Thinking

Task 1 Overview and Comprehension

Directions: *While you read an article, it is a good habit to take down some reading notes. Reading notes usually include the main idea and key information provided in the article. Please read through the text and provide the missing information in the following Reading Notes.*

Reading Notes	
What Is Known About the Birth of the First IVF Child in the World?	
Who Is Robert Edwards and What Is Known About His Research?	
What Are the Major Ethical Challenges According to the Text?	

Directions: *Some people think reproductive medicine has saved many women from despair and should be regarded as the most helpful medical technology in terms of facilitating the development of humankind while others criticize that reproductive medicine has destroyed the biological and social order and created many ethical challenges to human beings. Which position would you support? Please work in groups and conduct a debate in English in class.*

Topic	The pro: Reproductive medicine has a positive influence on human development and should be further promoted. The con: Reproductive medicine has a negative influence on human development and should be banned.
Steps	1. Thesis statement: One speaker from each group states the main thesis of his/her group (2 minutes). 2. Cross examination: Members from each group can raise questions to the other group (15 minutes). 3. Summary: One speaker from each group summarizes the main idea and concludes his/her argument (3 minutes). 4. The chair summarizes and comments on the debate (3 minutes).

Part 3 Extended Reading

Medical Professionalism in the New Millennium: A Physician Charter①

Preamble

Professionalism is the basis of medicine's contract with society. It demands placing the interests of patients above those of the physician, setting and maintaining standards of competence and **integrity**, and providing expert advice to society on matters of health.

At present, the medical profession is confronted by an **explosion** of technology, changing market forces, problems in health care delivery, **bioterrorism**, and globalization. As a result, physicians find it increasingly difficult to meet their responsibilities to patients and society. In these circumstances, reaffirming the fundamental and universal principles and values of medical professionalism, which remain ideals to be pursued by all physicians, becomes all the more important.

The medical profession everywhere is embedded in diverse cultures and national traditions, but its members share the role of healer, which has roots extending back to Hippocrates. Despite differences, common themes **emerge** and form the basis of this Charter in the form of three fundamental principles and as a set of definitive professional responsibilities.

New Expressions	
professionalism /prə'feʃənəlɪzəm/ *n.* 专业水平；专业素质 **integrity** /ɪn'tegrəti/ *n.* 诚实；正直；完整	**explosion** /ɪk'spləuʒn/ *n.* 突增；猛增；激增 **bioterrorism** /ˌbaɪə'terərɪzəm/ *n.* 生物恐怖主义 **emerge** /i'mɜːrdʒ/ *v.* 出现

---

① The text is adapted from the following source: Project of the ABIM Foundation, ACP-ASIM Foundation, and European Federation of Internal Medicine. 2002. Medical professionalism in the new millennium: A physician charter. *Annals of Internal Medicine, 136*(3): 243–246.

Fundamental Principles

Principle of **primacy** of patient welfare. This principle is based on a **dedication** to serving the interest of the patient. Altruism contributes to the trust that is central to the physician—patient relationship.

Principle of patient **autonomy.** Physicians must have respect for patient autonomy. Physicians must be honest with their patients and **empower** them to make informed decisions about their treatment.

Principle of social justice. The medical profession must promote justice in the health care system, including the fair distribution of health care resources.

A Set of Professional Responsibilities

Commitment to professional competence. Physicians must be committed to lifelong learning and be responsible for maintaining the medical knowledge and clinical and team skills necessary for the provision of quality care.

Commitment to honesty with patients. Physicians must ensure that patients are completely and honestly informed before they have consented to treatment and after treatment has occurred. This expectation does not mean that patients should be involved in every minute decision about medical care; rather, they must be empowered to decide on the course of therapy. Physicians should also acknowledge that in health care, medical errors that injure patients do sometimes occur. Whenever patients are injured as a consequence of medical care, patients should be informed promptly because failure to do so seriously **compromises** patient and societal trust.

Commitment to patient **confidentiality**. Earning the trust and confidence of patients requires that appropriate confidentiality safeguards be applied to disclosure of patient information. This commitment extends to discussions with persons acting on a patient's behalf when obtaining the patient's own consent is not feasible.

New Expressions

primacy /'praɪməsi/ *n.* 首要；至高无上

dedication /ˌdedɪ'keɪʃn/ *n.* 献身；奉献

autonomy /ɔː'tɑːnəmi/ *n.* 自主；自主权

empower /ɪm'paʊər/ *v.* 赋权

compromise /'kɑːmprəmaɪz/ *v.*（尤指因行为不很明智）使陷入危险；使受到怀疑

confidentiality /ˌkɑːnfɪˌdenʃi'æləti/ *n.* 保密性；机密性

Commitment to maintaining appropriate relations with patients. Given the **inherent vulnerability** and dependency of patients, certain relationships between physicians and patients must be avoided. In particular, physicians should never exploit patients for any sexual advantage, personal financial gain, or other private purpose.

Commitment to improving quality of care. Physicians must be dedicated to continuous improvement in the quality of health care. This commitment **entails** not only maintaining clinical competence but also working collaboratively with other professionals to reduce medical errors, increase patient safety, **minimize** overuse of health care resources, and **optimize** the outcomes of care.

Commitment to improving **access** to care. Medical professionalism demands that the objective of all health care systems be the **availability** of a **uniform** and adequate standard of care. Physicians must individually and collectively **strive** to reduce **barriers** to **equitable** health care.

Commitment to a just distribution of **finite** resources. While meeting the needs of individual patients, physicians are required to provide health care that is based on the wise and **cost-effective** management of limited clinical resources. They should be committed to working with other physicians, hospitals, and payers to develop guidelines for cost-effective care.

Commitment to scientific knowledge. Much of medicine's contract with society is based on the integrity and appropriate use of scientific knowledge and technology. Physicians have a duty to **uphold** scientific standards, to promote research, and to create new knowledge and ensure its appropriate use.

Commitment to maintaining trust by managing conflicts of interest. Medical professionals and their organizations have many opportunities to compromise their

New Expressions	
inherent /ɪn'hɪrənt/ *adj.* 固有的；内在的	**strive** /straɪv/ *v.* 努力；奋斗；力争；力求
vulnerability /ˌvʌlnərə'bɪləti/ *n.* 弱点	**barrier** /'bæriər/ *n.* 障碍；阻力
entail /ɪn'teɪl/ *v.* 牵涉；需要；使必要	**equitable** /'ekwɪtəbl/ *adj.* 公平合理的；公正的
minimize /'mɪnɪmaɪz/ *v.* 最小化	**finite** /'faɪnaɪt/ *adj.* 有限的；有限制的
optimize /'ɑːptɪmaɪz/ *v.* 使最优化；充分利用	**cost-effective** /ˌkɔːst ɪ'fektɪv/ *adj.* 有最佳利润的；有成本效益的；划算的
access /'ækses/ *n.* （使用或见到的）机会；权利	
availability /əˌveɪlə'bɪləti/ *n.* 可及性	**uphold** /ʌp'həʊld/ *v.* 支持；维持
uniform /'juːnɪfɔːrm/ *adj.* 一致的；统一的；一律的	

professional responsibilities by pursuing private gain or personal advantage. Physicians have an obligation to recognize, disclose to the general public, and deal with conflicts of interest that arise in the course of their professional duties and activities.

Commitment to professional responsibilities. As members of a profession, physicians are expected to work collaboratively to maximize patient care, be respectful of one another, and participate in the processes of self-regulation, including remediation and discipline of members who have failed to meet professional standards.

Summary

The practice of medicine in the modern era is beset with unprecedented challenges in virtually all cultures and societies. These challenges center on increasing disparities among the legitimate needs of patients, the available resources to meet those needs, the increasing dependence on market forces to transform health care systems, and the temptation for physicians to forsake their traditional commitment to the primacy of patients' interests. To maintain the fidelity of medicine's social contract during this turbulent time, we believe that physicians must reaffirm their active dedication to the principles of professionalism, which entails not only their personal commitment to the welfare of their patients but also collective efforts to improve the health care system for the welfare of society. This Charter is intended to encourage such dedication and to promote an action agenda for the profession of medicine that is universal in scope and purpose.

New Expressions

remediation /rɪˌmiːdi'eɪʃn/ *n.* 补救；纠正；（尤指对环境破坏的）整改，制止

beset /bɪ'set/ *v.* 困扰；威胁

unprecedented /ʌn'presɪdentɪd/ *adj.* 前所未有的；空前的；没有先例的

disparity /dɪ'spærəti/ *n.* （尤指因不公正对待引起的）不同，不等，差异，悬殊

temptation /temp'teɪʃn/ *n.* 引诱；诱惑

forsake /fər'seɪk/ *v.* 抛弃，遗弃，离开（尤指不履行责任）

fidelity /fɪ'deləti/ *n.* 忠诚；忠实；忠贞

turbulent /'tɜːrbjələnt/ *adj.* 动荡的；动乱的；骚动的；混乱的

Note

Preamble: 序言。这是《新世纪医师职业精神：医师宣言》的序言。1999 年，欧洲内科医学联盟（the European Federation of Internal Medicine）、美国医师协会 –

美国内科医学会基金会（ACP-ASIM Foundation, American College of Physicians-American Society of Internal Medicine Foundation）和美国内科学基金（ABIM Foundation, American Board of Internal Medicine Foundation）共同发起了医师职业精神项目。2002 年，《新世纪医师职业精神：医师宣言》英文版正式在《内科学年鉴》（*Annals of Internal Medicine*）和《柳叶刀》（*Lancet*）上发表。本文节选自发表于《内科学年鉴》上的原文。

Post-reading Activities

I **Speaking Practice: Oral Presentation**

Directions: *It is believed that physicians today worldwide are experiencing frustration as changes in the health care delivery systems in virtually all industrialized countries threaten the very nature and values of medical professionalism. Could you talk about what challenges physicians face in contemporary China and what suggestions you could offer to help physicians to cope with the problems?*

II **Reflective Writing Practice: Mini-research Project**

Directions: *Based on your reading and discussion, please follow the given steps and conduct a small-scale research project on ideal physicians in China with your group members. Complete the following Research Report by filling out your major findings. Then reflect on your findings and write a short essay entitled "Ideal Physicians in China". The word limit is suggested to be 150–200 words.*

Research Report	
Research Objective	To investigate the qualities of ideal physicians in China
Research Method	Interview
Research Procedures	1. Search and read literature on ideal physicians. 2. Design an interview outline for deeper investigation of qualities ideal physicians should possess in China. 3. Conduct interviews to at least five individuals. 4. Analyze the interview data.

Research Report	
Research Findings	Please summarize the findings based on your data analysis. You can summarize the qualities described by the interviewees in line with the principles mentioned in the Physician Charter.

Unit 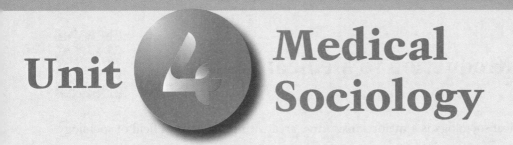 Medical Sociology

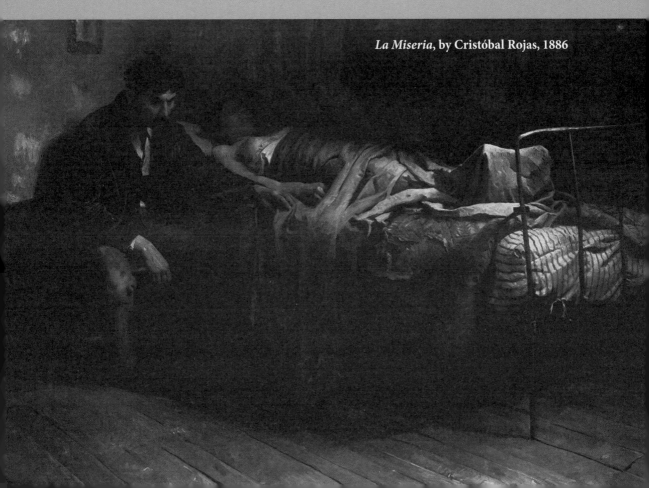

La Miseria, by Cristóbal Rojas, 1886

Part 1 Academic Horizon

An Introduction to Medical Sociology[①]

Medical sociology is a major **substantive** area within the general field of sociology. As an academic discipline, sociology is concerned with the social causes and consequences of human behavior. Thus, it follows that medical sociology focuses on the social causes and consequences of health and illness. Medical sociology brings sociological perspectives, theories, and methods to the study of health, illness, medical practice, and policy. Areas of **investigation** include the social causes of health and disease, health disparities, the social behavior of health care **personnel** and their patients, the social functions of health organizations and institutions, the social patterns of the **utilization** of health services, social policies toward health, and similar topics. What makes medical sociology important is the critical role social factors play in determining or influencing health outcomes.

A major development in the study of health and disease is the growing recognition of the relevance of social determinants. The term "social determinants of health" refers to social practices and conditions (such as lifestyles, living and work situations), class position (income, education, and occupation), stressful circumstances, poverty, and economic (e.g. unemployment, business **recessions**), political (e.g. policies, government benefits), and religious factors that affect the health of individuals, groups, and communities, either positively or negatively. Social determinants not only **foster** illness

New Expressions	
substantive /ˈsʌbstəntɪv/ *adj.* 实质性的；本质上的；重大的；严肃认真的	体人员，职员
investigation /ɪnˌvestɪˈɡeɪʃn/ *n.* 科学研究；学术研究	**utilization** /ˌjuːtələˈzeɪʃn/ *n.* 使用；利用；应用
personnel /ˌpɜːrsəˈnel/ *n.*（组织或军队中的）全	**recession** /rɪˈseʃn/ *n.* 经济衰退；经济萎缩
	foster /ˈfɑːstər/ *v.* 促进；助长；培养；鼓励

① The text is adapted from the following sources: Cockerham, W. C. 2016. *Medical Sociology* (13th ed.). London: Routledge.

Schaefer, R. T. 2015. *Sociology: A Brief Introduction* (11th ed.). New York: McGraw-Hill Education.

 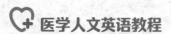

and disability, they also **enhance** prospects for coping with or preventing disease and maintaining health. Once thought of as secondary or distant influences on health and disease, it now appears that social connections can be a fundamental cause of health problems. The social context of a person's life determines the risk of exposure, the **susceptibility** to a disease, and the course and outcome of the **affliction**—regardless of whether it is **infectious**, genetic, **metabolic**, **malignant**, or **degenerative**. Thus, it can be claimed that "society may indeed make you sick or **conversely** promote your health".

For example, in addressing the question of whether or not social factors matter to health, the National Research Council and the Institute of Medicine **documented** various links between social determinants and health. The most important social factors determining health were found to be income, **accumulated** wealth, education, occupational characteristics, and social inequality based on race and ethnic groups. These variables have direct effects on both unhealthy and healthy lifestyles, high or low risk health behavior, and on living conditions, food security, levels of stresses and **strains**, social disadvantages over the life course, environmental factors that influence biological outcomes through gene expression, and other connections.

Social factors are also important in influencing the manner in which societies organize their resources to cope with health **hazards** and deliver health care to the population at large. Individuals, groups, and societies typically respond to health problems in a manner consistent with their culture, norms, and values. Social and political values influence the choices made, institutions formed, and levels of funding provided for health. It is no accident that the United States has its particular form of health care delivery and other nations have their own approaches. Health is not simply a matter of biology but involves a number of factors that are cultural, political, economic, and—especially—social in nature.

New Expressions	
enhance /ɪnˈhæns/ v. 提高；增强；增进	**degenerative** /dɪˈdʒenərətɪv/ adj. （随着时间的推移）变性的，退行性的
susceptibility /səˌseptəˈbɪləti/ n. 易受影响（或伤害等）的特性；敏感性；过敏性	**conversely** /ˈkɑːnvɜːrsli/ adv. 相反地；反过来
affliction /əˈflɪkʃn/ n. 折磨；痛苦	**document** /ˈdɑːkjument/ v. 记录，记载（详情）
infectious /ɪnˈfekʃəs/ adj. 传染性的，感染的（尤指通过呼吸）	**accumulated** /əˈkjuːmjəleɪtɪd/ adj. 累积的
metabolic /ˌmetəˈbɑːlɪk/ adj. 新陈代谢的	**strain** /streɪn/ n. 压力；重负；重压之下出现的问题（或担忧等）
malignant /məˈlɪɡnənt/ adj. 恶性的	**hazard** /ˈhæzərd/ n. 危险；危害

The earliest works in medical sociology were undertaken by physicians and not by sociologists who tended to ignore the field. The term "medical sociology" first appeared in 1894, in a medical article by Charles McIntire on the importance of social factors in health. Other early work by physicians included essays on the relationship between medicine and society in 1902 by Elizabeth Blackwell, the first woman to graduate from an American medical school (Geneva Medical College in New York), and James Warbasse who wrote a book in 1909 called *Medical Sociology* about physicians as a unique social class. Warbasse also organized a Section on Sociology for the American Public Health Association in 1909 that lacked sociologists and was **comprised** almost entirely of physicians and social workers.

It remained for Michael Davis and Bernard Stern to publish books on health with a sociological perspective. Davis published *Immigrant Health and the Community* in 1921 and Stern's book appeared in 1927, titled *Social Factors in Medical Progress*. A few publications followed in the 1930s, such as Lawrence Henderson's 1935 paper on the physician and patient as a social system that **subsequently** influenced **Talcott Parsons**[1] important **conceptualization** of the sick role years later. Henderson was a physician and **biochemist** at Harvard, who became interested in sociological theory and changed careers to teach in the new sociology department when it was formed in the early 1930s. Parsons was one of his students.

The appearance, in 1951, of Talcott Parsons' book *The Social System*, oriented American medical sociology toward theory. This book, written to explain a relatively complex **structural functionalist**[2] model of society, in which social systems are linked to corresponding systems of personality and culture, contained Parsons' concept of the sick role. Unlike other major social theorists preceding him, Parsons formulated an analysis of the function of medicine in society. Parsons presented an ideal representation of how people in Western society act when sick.

People who are considered sick are **exempted** from their normal, day-to-day responsibilities and generally do not suffer blame for their condition. Yet they are obligated to try to get well, which includes seeking competent professional care. The

---

New Expressions

comprise /kəm'praɪz/ *v.* 包括；包含；由……组成

subsequently /'sʌbsɪkwəntli/ *adv.* 随后；后来；之后；接着

conceptualization /kənˌseptʃuəlaɪ'zeɪʃn/ *n.* 概念化

biochemist /ˌbaɪou'kemɪst/ *n.* 生物化学家

exempt /ɪg'zempt/ *v.* 免除；豁免

医学人文英语教程

merit of the concept is that it describes a patterned set of expectations defining the norms and values appropriate to being sick, for both the sick person and others who **interact with** that person. Parsons also pointed out that physicians are invested by society with the function of social control, similar to the role provided by priests and the police, to serve as a means to control **deviance**. Physicians verify a patient's condition either as "illness" or as "recovered". The ill person becomes dependent on the physician, because the latter can control valued rewards (not only treatment of illness, but also excused absences from work and school). Parsons suggests that the physician-patient relationship is somewhat like that between parent and child. Like a parent, the physician helps the patient to enter society as a full and functioning adult. In the case of the sick role, illness is the deviance, and its undesirable nature **reinforces** the motivation to be healthy.

However, this was not the case, as Parsons' model was severely criticized and his views are no longer widely accepted. Nevertheless, he provided a theoretical approach for medical sociology that brought the subdiscipline the intellectual recognition it needed in its early development in the United States. This is because the institutional support for sociology in America was in universities, where the discipline was established more **firmly** than elsewhere in the world. Without academic **legitimacy** and the subsequent participation of such well-known, mainstream academic sociologists in the 1960s, such as Robert Merton and Erving Goffman, medical sociology would lack the early professional **credentials** and **stature** it currently has in both academic and applied settings. Parsons' views on society may not be the **optimal paradigm** for explaining illness, but Parsons was important in the emergence of medical sociology as an academic field.

New Expressions	
interact with 与……互动	**credentials** /krə'denʃlz/ *n.* 资格；资历
deviance /'diːvɪəns/ *n.* 不正常；异常；偏离常轨	**stature** /'stætʃər/ *n.* 名望；声望
reinforce /ˌriːɪn'fɔːrs/ *v.* 加强；充实；使更强烈	**optimal** /'ɑːptɪməl/ *adj.* 最佳的；最适宜的
firmly /'fɜːrmli/ *adv.* 坚定地；坚固地	**paradigm** /'pærədaɪm/ *n.* 范式；范例；典范；样式
legitimacy /lɪ'dʒɪtɪməsi/ *n.* 合法性；合理性	

Notes

1. Talcott Parsons: 塔尔科特·帕森斯，1902—1979；美国著名社会学家，以其社会行动理论和结构功能主义而闻名。帕森斯被认为是 20 世纪社会学界最有影响力的人物之一，是医学社会学发展的重要人物。帕森斯在《社会系统》（ *The Social System* ）一书中提出了社会学第一个分析健康和疾病在社会生活中的作用的重要理论。在这一理论中，帕森斯认为，如果有太多的人声称自己生病，那么这将使社会产生失调，因此需要对"病人角色"的进入进行规范。Parsons was best known for his social action theory and structural functionalism. The first major theory within sociology that analyzed the role of health and illness in social life was devised in his book *The Social System*. In this theory, Parsons argued that if too many people claimed to be ill, then this would have a dysfunctional impact on society, and therefore entry into the "sick role" needed to be regulated.

2. **structural functionalist**: 结构功能主义的。Structural functionalism is a framework for building theory that sees society as a complex system whose parts work together to promote solidarity and stability.

Post-reading Activities

I **Speaking Practice: Group Discussion**

Directions: *Please discuss the following questions in small groups. After your discussion, please share your opinions with the whole class.*

1. Based on your reading, what have you learned about medical sociology?
2. What are the social determinants of health based on your daily life experiences?

II **Speaking Practice: Oral Presentation**

Directions: *The following sociologists mentioned in the text have made great contributions to the development of sociology. Choose one figure and search for more information on the Internet. Then give an oral presentation to introduce the biography and achievements of the figure to the whole class.*

| Talcott Parsons | Robert Merton | Erving Goffman |

Part 2 Thematic Reading

Medicalization[1]

Implicit in Parsons' concept of sickness as a form of deviance is the idea that medicine is (and should be) an institution for the social control of deviant behaviors. That is, it is medicine's task to control abnormal behavior by medical means on behalf of society. However, some medical sociologists have expressed concern that medicine has taken responsibility for an ever greater proportion of deviant behaviors and bodily conditions by defining them as medical problems. Acts that might have been defined as **sin** or crime and controlled by the church or the law are increasingly regarded as illnesses to be controlled through medical treatment, as are certain physical differences like short **stature**, small female **breasts**, and male **baldness**. This trend is known as "medicalization" and occurs when non-medical problems are defined as problems that need to be treated medically, usually as an illness or disorder of some type. "Medicalization," according to Joseph Davis, "is the name for the process by which medical definitions and practices are applied to behaviors, psychological phenomena, and **somatic** experiences not previously within the conceptual or therapeutic scope of medicine." As Thomas Szasz put it, "with increasing **zeal**, physicians and especially **psychiatrists** began to call 'illness'... anything and everything in which they could detect any sign of malfunctioning, based on no matter what the norm."

These comments call attention to the trend toward making sickness and deviance

New Expressions	
medicalization /ˌmedɪkələɪˈzeɪʃn/ *n.* 医学化	**baldness** /ˈbɔːldnəs/ *n.* 秃顶；秃头
implicit /ɪmˈplɪsɪt/ *adj.* 成为一部分的；内含的	**somatic** /soʊˈmætɪk/ *adj.* 躯体的
sin /sɪn/ *n.* 罪，罪恶，罪过（对神的冒犯或对宗教戒律、道德规范的违犯）	**zeal** /ziːl/ *n.* 热情；激情
stature /ˈstætʃər/ *n.* 身高；个子	**psychiatrist** /saɪˈkaɪətrɪst/ *n.* 精神科医生；精神病学家
breast /brest/ *n.* （女子的）乳房	

---

[1] The text is adapted from the following source: Cockerham, W. C. 2016. *Medical Sociology* (13th ed.). London: Routledge.

not only **synonymous** but also toward treating deviance exclusively in a medical mode. Rick Mayes and Allan Horwitz observed that the *American Psychiatric Association's Diagnostic and Statistical Manual of Mental Disorders* first published in 1952 listed 106 mental disorders and was 130 pages in length. The fourth edition published in 1994 and revised in 2000 had 297 disorders and consisted of 886 pages, while the fifth edition released in 2013 has 341 disorders and 992 pages. Clearly, there has been **proliferation** of diagnoses in psychiatry, including problems, such as "oppositional defiant disorder" (defiant acts by children, such as losing **tempers** or being **annoying**, angry, or **spiteful**) that would appear to be **dubious** without evidence of other more abnormal behavior and others such as "**binge** eating disorder" and "**cannabis** withdrawal" that arguably have questionable **validity** as a mental disorder. "Disorder of written expression" (bad writing) was fortunately removed from DSM-5. Some critics, such as Andrew Twaddle, have gone so far as to claim that "there are few, if any, problems of human behavior that some group does not think of as medical problems". Freidson has likewise argued that medicine has established **jurisdiction** far wider than justified by its **demonstrable** capacity to "cure".

Nonetheless, the medical profession has been successful in gaining authority to define **aberrant** behaviors and even naturally occurring physical conditions, such as aging as illness problems best handled by the physician. For example, **hyperactivity** at school by children is defined as **Attention-Deficit/Hyperactivity Disorder** (ADHD) and requires **Ritalin**; **menopause** is treated with **estrogen** replacement therapy, whose side effects were determined a few years later to promote even greater risk from blood

---

New Expressions

synonymous /sɪ'nɑːnɪməs/ *adj.* 同义的

mental disorder 精神障碍

proliferation /prəˌlɪfə'reɪʃn/ *n.* 激增；增殖；增生

temper /'tempər/ *n.* 脾气；易怒的性情

annoying /ə'nɔɪɪŋ/ *adj.* 使恼怒的；使生气的；使烦恼的

spiteful /'spaɪtfl/ *adj.* 恶意的；居心不良的；故意使人苦恼的

dubious /'duːbɪəs/ *adj.* 怀疑的；无把握的；拿不准的

binge /bɪndʒ/ *n.* 大吃大喝

cannabis /'kænəbɪs/ *n.* 大麻制品

validity /və'lɪdəti/ *n.* （法律上的）有效，合法性；（正式的）认可

jurisdiction /ˌdʒʊrɪs'dɪkʃn/ *n.* 管辖区域；管辖范围

demonstrable /dɪ'mɑːnstrəbl/ *adj.* 明显的；可表明的；可论证的；可证明的

aberrant /æ'berənt/ *adj.* 违反常规的；反常的；异常的

hyperactivity /ˌhaɪpəræk'tɪvəti/ *n.* 过分活跃；多动

Attention-Deficit/Hyperactivity Disorder 注意力缺陷 / 多动障碍

Ritalin /'rɪtəlɪn/ *n.* 利他林（中枢兴奋药）

menopause /'menəpɔːz/ *n.* 绝经期；（妇女的）更年期

estrogen /'estrədʒən/ *n.* 雌激素

clots, stroke, heart disease, and breast cancer; being short in stature necessitates growth **hormones** for the person afflicted with below average height; and male baldness is slowed or prevented by using **Propecia** and lost hair is restored by surgical transplants. There was a time when hyperactivity, menopause, shortness, and baldness were not medical conditions. A similar trend is seen in studies of mental health showing psychiatry transforming normal **sorrow** into clinically treated depression and natural anxiety into an anxiety disorder.

Of course, for some people, new medical treatments for previously untreated conditions can be positive, such as the development of **Viagra** and similar drugs for **erectile** dysfunction. However, current accounts of medicalization describe an even greater **expansion** of this process. This outcome has led Adele Clarke and her colleagues to declare that the growth of medical jurisdiction over social problems is "one of the most **potent** transformations of the last half of the 20th century in the West". Whereas medicalization has traditionally been a means by which professional medicine acquired increasingly more problems to treat, Clarke and her colleagues suggest that major technological and scientific advances in biomedicine are taking this capability even further and producing what she and her colleagues refer to as "biomedicalization". Biomedicalization consists of the capability of computer information and new technologies to extend medical **surveillance** and treatment interventions well beyond past boundaries, by the use of genetics, **bioengineering**, chemoprevention, individualized drugs, multiple sources of information, patient data banks, **digitalized** patient records, and other innovations. Also important in this process is the Internet, advertising, **consumerism**, and the role of **pharmaceutical** companies in marketing their products.

New Expressions

clot /klɑːt/ *n.* 血块

hormone /ˈhɔːrmoʊn/ *n.* 激素；荷尔蒙

Propecia /prəˈpesiə/ *n.* 非那雄胺（生发剂）

sorrow /ˈsɑːroʊ/ *n.* 悲伤；悲痛；悲哀

Viagra /vaɪˈægrə/ *n.* 万艾可（壮阳药）

erectile /ɪˈrektaɪl/ *adj.* （身体部位）能勃起的

expansion /ɪkˈspænʃn/ *n.* 扩张；扩展；扩大；膨胀

potent /ˈpoʊtnt/ *adj.* 有强效的；有力的；烈性的；影响身心的

surveillance /sɜːrˈveɪləns/ *n.* （对犯罪嫌疑人或可能发生犯罪的地方的）监视

bioengineering /ˌbaɪoʊˌendʒɪˈnɪrɪŋ/ *n.* 生物工程

digitalized /ˈdɪdʒɪtəlaɪzd/ *adj.* 数字化的

consumerism /kənˈsuːmərɪzəm/ *n.* 消费；消费主义

pharmaceutical /ˌfɑːrməˈsuːtɪkl/ *adj.* 制药的；配药的；卖药的

The increasing **commercialization** of health products and services in the expansion of the medical marketplace has been noted by other medical sociologists. Peter Conrad and Valerie Leiter observe that insurance companies can **counteract** medicalization by restricting access, but there are other forces **facilitating** the process. Conrad finds that the engines pushing medicalization have changed, with biotechnology, consumers, and managed care now being the driving forces. "Doctors," Conrad states, "are still the gatekeepers for medical treatment, but their role is more **subordinate** in the expansion or contraction of medicalization." He notes that biotechnology has long been associated with medicalization, and the pharmaceutical industry is playing an increasingly central role in promoting its products directly to consumers, while in the future the **impact** of genetics may be substantial. Already, we have seen the use of the term "pharmaceuticalization of society" to describe the growth of the drug markets internationally through large-scale advertising **campaigns** directed to both physicians and the public at large, including drugs for non-medical (enhancement) purposes.

In the meantime, consumers have become major players in the health marketplace through their purchase of health insurance plans, health products, and the like, and their demand for these products also **fuels** medicalization. The Internet, in particular, has led to easier consumer access to health-related goods. Managed care, in turn, has become the **dominant** form of health care delivery in the United States, which makes insurance companies as third-party payers important in both **bolstering** medicalization through its coverage of particular services and a **constraint** in placing limitations on those services. Thus managed care plays an important role in the medicalization process. Although medicalization is prevalent in the United States, observes Conrad, it is increasingly an international phenomenon with multinational drug companies leading the way. While

New Expressions	
commercialization /kə͵mɜːrʃlə'zeɪʃn/ *n.* 商品化；商业化	**campaign** /kæm'peɪn/ *n.* 运动（为社会、商业或政治目的而进行的一系列有计划的活动）
counteract /͵kaʊntər'ækt/ *v.* 抵制；抵消；抵抗	**fuel** /'fjuːəl/ *v.* 增加；加强；刺激
facilitate /fə'sɪlɪteɪt/ *v.* 促进；促使；使便利	**dominant** /'dɑːmɪnənt/ *adj.* 首要的；占支配地位的；占优势的；显著的
subordinate /sə'bɔːrdɪnət/ *adj.* 隶属的；从属的；下级的	**bolster** /'boʊlstər/ *v.* 改善；加强
impact /'ɪmpækt/ *n.* 巨大影响；强大作用	**constraint** /kən'streɪnt/ *n.* 限制；限定；约束

public and professional medical concern about medicalization may be growing, the process it represents is still a powerful influence on behavior and our understanding of it has its origins in Parsons' work.

Post-reading Activities

I Language Building-up

Task 1 Extensive Vocabulary Enlargement

Directions: *The following words are taken from the text. Please follow the three-step learning in this part and build up your own Extensive Vocabulary Chart.*

Step 1. Read through the words and underline them in the text. Circle the ones that are particularly new to you. Look up the words in the dictionary and put the equivalent Chinese translation in the chart below.

Step 2. While you go back to the text, please feel free to put any other words into the blanks provided in the extra lines in the chart.

Extensive Vocabulary Chart				
medicalization	sin	baldness	somatic	psychiatrist
synonymous	mental	proliferation	spiteful	validity
hyperactivity	menopause	hormone	expansion	bioengineering
digitalized	pharmaceutical	subordinate	campaign	constraint

Step 3. Please group the above words based on their parts of speech and meanings.

Nouns	
Verbs	
Adjectives	
Adverbs and Prepositions	
Medical Terminology	
Terminology in Other Fields	

Task 2　Intensive Vocabulary Enhancement

Directions: *The following 10 words are chosen from the text. They will form the intensive vocabulary in this unit. For intensive vocabulary, you are supposed to be able to explain them in English and use them in sentence and discourse constructions.*

Step 1. Please read through the words and be familiar with their Chinese and English definitions. Recall where and how they are used in the text.

No.	Word	Translation	Definition	Status
			Intensive Vocabulary Chart	
1	implicit	成为一部分的；内含的	*adj.* forming part of sth. (although perhaps not directly expressed)	☆ ☆ ☆ ☆ ☆
2	stature	身高；个子	*n.* a person's height	☆ ☆ ☆ ☆ ☆

(Continued)

			Intensive Vocabulary Chart	
No.	Word	Translation	Definition	Status
3	zeal	热情；激情	*n.* great energy or enthusiasm connected with sth. that you feel strongly about	☆ ☆ ☆ ☆ ☆
4	dubious	怀疑的；无把握的；拿不准的	*adj.* not certain and slightly suspicious about sth.; not knowing whether sth. is good or bad	☆ ☆ ☆ ☆ ☆
5	aberrant	违反常规的；反常的；异常的	*adj.* not usual or not socially acceptable	☆ ☆ ☆ ☆ ☆
6	potent	有强效的；有力的；烈性的；影响身心的	*adj.* powerful	☆ ☆ ☆ ☆ ☆
7	surveillance	（对犯罪嫌疑人或可能发生犯罪的地方的）监视	*n.* the act of carefully watching a person suspected of a crime or a place where a crime may be committed	☆ ☆ ☆ ☆ ☆
8	counteract	抵制；抵消；抵抗	*v.* to do sth. to reduce or prevent the bad or harmful effects of sth.	☆ ☆ ☆ ☆ ☆
9	fuel	增加；加强；刺激	*v.* to increase sth.; to make sth. stronger	☆ ☆ ☆ ☆ ☆
10	dominant	首要的；占支配地位的；占优势的；显著的	*adj.* more important, powerful or noticeable than other things	☆ ☆ ☆ ☆ ☆

Step 2. Please tick the status for each word based on your own situation. If one word is very new or difficult for you, please tick five stars. Likewise, if one word is comparatively easy for you and you don't have to spend too much time on reading and learning it, then tick one star. The number of stars represents the difficulty of commanding a word in your eyes.

Step 3. Please complete the following 10 sentences by choosing appropriate words from the Intensive Vocabulary Chart. Please change the forms of the words where necessary.

1. He had an absolute _____ for litigation.
   他对诉讼有着极大的热情。

2. The ability to listen is _____ in the teacher's role.
   教师的角色包含了倾听的能力。

3. Passion is a force so _____ that people would still remember it long after it has faded away.

热情是一种如此强大的力量，以至人们在它消失了很长时间后仍然会将它铭记于心。

4. The police are keeping the suspects under constant _____.

警方正对嫌疑人实施不间断监视。

5. These exercises aim to _____ the effects of stress and tension.

这些训练旨在抵消压力与紧张带来的影响。

6. The firm has achieved a(n) _____ position in the world market.

这家公司在国际市场上占有举足轻重的地位。

7. It's more than his physical _____ that makes him remarkable.

他的与众不同之处不只是在于他的身高。

8. I was rather _____ about the whole idea.

我对这整个想法很怀疑。

9. The doctor tries to find the cause of the child's _____ behavior.

医生试图找到这个孩子反常行为的原因。

10. Higher salaries may help to _____ inflation.

工资的提高有可能会刺激通货膨胀。

Task 3   Expressions and Sentences

Directions: *The following sentences are taken from the text. In each sentence, there are one or two phrases being underlined. Please refer to the dictionary and write down the explanation of the phrases in the line entitled "Meaning Exploration". After that, please choose one phrase and make a sentence with it. Write the sentence in the line entitled "Sentence Making".*

Sentence 1

Original Sentence	... medicine has taken responsibility for an ever greater proportion of deviant behaviors and bodily conditions by defining them as medical problems.
Meaning Exploration	*take responsibility for:* *define (sth.) as:*
Sentence Making	

Sentence 2

Original Sentence	These comments call attention to the trend toward making sickness and deviance not only synonymous but also toward treating deviance exclusively in a medical mode.
Meaning Exploration	*call attention to:*
Sentence Making	

Sentence 3

Original Sentence	... being short in stature necessitates growth hormones for the person afflicted with below average height...
Meaning Exploration	*(be) afflicted with:*
Sentence Making	

Sentence 4

Original Sentence	... through large-scale advertising campaigns directed to both physicians and the public at large, including drugs for non-medical (enhancement) purposes.
Meaning Exploration	*at large:*
Sentence Making	

Sentence 5

Original Sentence	Although medicalization is prevalent in the United States, observes Conrad, it is increasingly an international phenomenon with multinational drug companies leading the way.
Meaning Exploration	*be prevalent in:* *lead the way:*
Sentence Making	

II   Critical Reading and Thinking

Task 1   Overview and Comprehension

Directions: *Please summarize the main idea of the text by filling out the information in the table below.*

Summary of the Main Content	
Origin of Medicalization	
Definition of Medicalization	
Origin of Biomedicalization	
Definition of Biomedicalization	

Task 2   Reflection and Discussion

Directions: *After reading, please reflect on the theme of the text. Work in groups and share your opinions on the following questions with other group members.*

1. Have you observed some phenomenon of medicalization in your daily life? Please describe the details.
2. Why does managed care play an important role in the medicalization process in the United States?
3. What would be the social consequences of medicalization?
4. What is the role of commercialization of health products and services in medicalization?

Part 3　Extended Reading

Stigma[①]

Stigma refers to physical or social characteristics that are identified as **demeaning** or are socially disapproved of, bringing **opprobrium**, social distance, or **discrimination**. Sociological studies of stigma and processes of **stigmatization** have been conducted largely within the **symbolic interactionist**[1] tradition from the 1960s onwards. Some early work, such as that of Goffman, theorized how stigmatizing processes work to produce discrimination and also investigated how the stigmatized person responds. For Goffman, there are some important differences depending on the type of stigma, which **governs** the extent to which people can manage their **self-identity** and protect their sense of self. Another source of ideas on stigma came from the disabled people's movement. An important early challenge to the individual model of disability was Paul Hunt's *Stigma: The Experience of Disability*. Hunt argued that, rather than disabled people's problems being seen as **arising from** their **impairments**, it was interactions between disabled people and able-bodied people that led to the stigmatizing of disability. In more recent times the concept has been successfully used to explore the situation of people with **HIV/AIDS**[2] and other health-related conditions.

The most successful and systematic account of the production of stigma is that

New Expressions	
stigma /'stɪgmə/ *n.* 耻辱；羞耻；污名	**stigmatization** /ˌstɪgmətə'zeɪʃn/ *n.* 污名化
demeaning /dɪ'miːnɪŋ/ *adj.* 降低身份的；失去尊严的	**govern** /'gʌvərn/ *v.* 控制；影响
opprobrium /ə'proʊbriəm/ *n.*（众人的）谴责，责难，抨击	**self-identity** /ˌself aɪ'dentəti/ *n.* 自我认同
	arise from 由……引起；起因于
discrimination /dɪˌskrɪmɪ'neɪʃn/ *n.* 区别对待；歧视；偏袒	**impairment** /ɪm'peəmənt/ *n.*（身体或智力方面的）缺陷，障碍，损伤；某种缺陷

①　The text is adapted from the following sources: Giddens, A. & Sutton, P. W. 2017. *Essential Concepts in Sociology* (2nd ed.). Cambridge: Polity Press.

Samari, E. et al. 2022. Perceived mental illness stigma among family and friends of young people with depression and its role in help-seeking: A qualitative inquiry. *BMC Psychiatry*, (22): 107.

of Erving Goffman. Goffman's work is an excellent example of the close linkage between social identity and **embodiment**, as he shows how some physical aspects of a person's body can present problems once these have been categorized by others as sources of stigma. He shows, for example, how disabled people can be stigmatized on the basis of readily observable physical impairments. Nonetheless, not all sources of stigma are physical, as stigma can **reside** in biographical features, character "**flaws**" or personal relationships. Stigma can take many forms. Physical stigma, such as a **visible** impairment, can often be hard or impossible to hide from others, and Goffman argues this can make the management of identities more difficult. Where this is the case, we can refer to a "**discredited**" stigma—one that has to be acknowledged in interactions. Biographical stigma, such as a previous criminal **conviction**, can be easier to hide from others, and in this case we can speak of a "discrediting" stigma—one that may lead to stigmatizing should it become more widely known. Managing this type may be somewhat easier, but it does still have to be continually controlled. A character stigma, such as associating with drug users, may also be a discrediting stigma, but it may turn into a discredited stigma if the person is observed with the wrong crowd. Note that Goffman is not suggesting people should hide stigma; he is just trying to make sense of how the process of stigmatization works in the real world and how people use strategies to avoid becoming stigmatized.

Goffman argued that stigma is a social relationship of **devaluation** in which one individual is **disqualified** from full social acceptance by others. Stigmatization often appears in a medical context as people become ill and their identity is changed—sometimes **temporarily**, but at other times, such as with chronic illnesses, **permanently**. Goffman argued that inherent in the process of stigmatization is social control. Stigmatizing groups is one way in which society at large controls their behavior. In some

New Expressions

embodiment /ɪmˈbɑːdɪmənt/ n.（体现一种思想或品质的）典型，化身

reside /rɪˈzaɪd/ v. 在于；由……造成（或引起）

flaw /flɔː/ n.（性格上的）弱点，缺点

visible /ˈvɪzəbl/ adj. 看得见的；可见的

discredited /dɪsˈkredɪtɪd/ adj. 不足信的；不名誉的

conviction /kənˈvɪkʃn/ n. 判罪；定罪

devaluation /ˌdiːˌvæljuˈeɪʃn/ n.（货币）贬值

disqualify /dɪsˈkwɑːlɪfaɪ/ v. 使不合格；使不适合；取消（某人）的资格

temporarily /ˌtempəˈrerəli/ adv. 短暂地；暂时地；临时地

permanently /ˈpɜːrmənəntli/ adv. 永久地；永恒地；长久地

cases, the stigma is never removed and the person is never fully accepted into society.

Stigma is a distinctive feature associated with mental illness. Sigma of mental illness can create social distance or rejection in the form of decrease in opportunity for employment, resulting from negative labels placed on people with mental illness (e.g. unstable, dangerous, and unpredictable), and fear of them. Consequently, such stigma can discourage individuals from seeking treatment due to the anticipation of being labeled with a mental illness and being discriminated against. Prior research has shown that family members of those with mental illness experience associated stigma with its negative consequences. Research showed that family members with severe mental illness experienced social **exclusion**, isolation and received nasty comments that devalue and ridicule them due to their mentally ill family members. Importantly, the research found that some family members tried to cope with the stigma by **concealing** mental illness from others to avoid discrimination, or by reducing contact with others to avoid being confronted with stigmatizing reactions. Reactions and coping styles from families can in turn have **implications** on the way individuals with mental illness cope with their illness.

New Expressions

exclusion /ɪkˈskluːʒn/ *n.* 排斥；排除在外
conceal /kənˈsiːl/ *v.* 隐藏；隐瞒；掩盖

implication /ˌɪmplɪˈkeɪʃn/ *n.* 可能的影响（或作用、结果）

Notes

1. **symbolic interactionist:** 符号互动论。It is a sociological perspective which holds that people act toward things based on the meaning those things have for them, and these meanings are derived from social interaction and modified through interpretation.

2. **HIV/AIDS:** HIV 指的是人体免疫缺损病毒，即艾滋病病毒，其英文全称为 human immunodeficiency virus。AIDS 指的是获得性免疫缺陷综合征，或称后天免疫缺乏综合征，即艾滋病，其英文全称为 Acquired Immune Deficiency Syndrome。

Post-reading Activities

I Speaking Practice: Interview

Directions: *Please work in pairs. Imagine one of you is an interviewee, a professor of medical sociology, and the other is an interviewer who interviews the professor about the concept of stigma. Please design three interview questions and take turns to be the interviewer and the interviewee.*

Interview questions:

1. _____
2. _____
3. _____

II Reflective Writing Practice: Mini-research Project

Directions: *Based on your reading and discussion, please follow the given steps and conduct a small-scale research project on mental illness stigma on campus with your group members. Complete the following Research Report by filling out your major findings. Then reflect on your findings and write a short essay entitled "Mental Illness Stigma on Campus". The word limit is suggested to be 150–200 words.*

Research Report	
Research Objectives	To investigate the current status of mental illness stigma on campus To find out strategies to help patients cope with mental illness stigma
Research Method	Questionnaire
Research Procedures	1. Search and read literature on mental illness stigma. 2. Design a questionnaire in reference to the prior literature and in response to your research objectives. 3. Send at least 30 questionnaires to students in your university. 4. Collect the questionnaires. 5. Analyze the data.

(Continued)

	Research Report
Research Findings	Please summarize the findings based on your data analysis and present the results of the questionnaires in response to the two research objectives. Current status: Coping strategies:

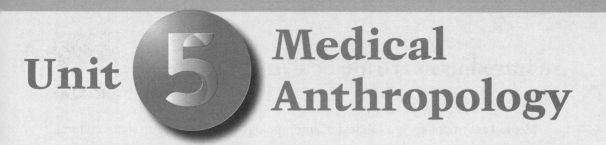

Unit 5 Medical Anthropology

A new language is proposed for examining the relationships among biology, experience, and meaning in the social construction of sickness as a phenomenon of everyday world.
—Arthur Kleinman

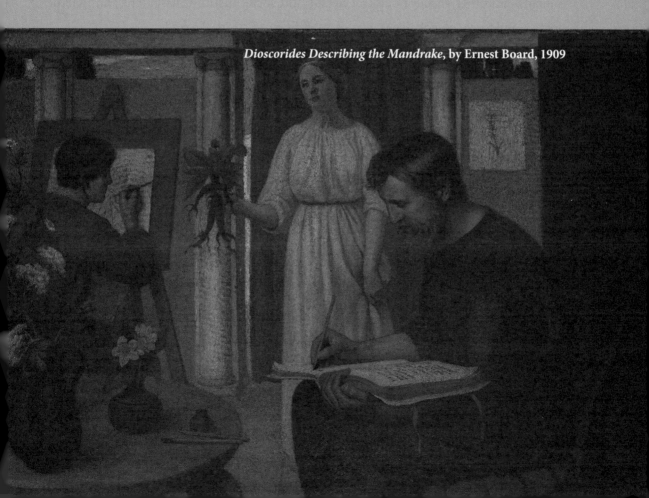

Dioscorides Describing the Mandrake, by Ernest Board, 1909

Part 1 Academic Horizon

An Introduction to Medical Anthropology[①]

Medical anthropology is a subfield of anthropology that **draws upon** social cultural, biological, and **linguistic** anthropology to better understand those factors which influence health and well-being, the experience and distribution of illness, the prevention and treatment of sickness, healing processes, the social relations of therapy management, and the cultural importance and utilization of **pluralistic** medical systems.

The discipline of medical anthropology draws upon many different theoretical approaches. It is as **attentive** to popular health culture as bio-scientific epidemiology, and the social construction of knowledge and politics of science as scientific discovery and **hypothesis** testing. Medical anthropologists examine how the health of individuals, larger social formations, and the environment are affected by interrelationships between humans and other species; cultural norms and social institutions; micro and macro politics; and forces of globalization as each of these affects local worlds.

Medical anthropology emerged as a special field of research and training after World War Ⅱ, when senior American anthropologists were brought in as **consultants** on health care projects in Latin America, Asia, and Africa. In the "Cold War" **rhetoric** of the time, aid to friendly "Third World countries" would **strengthen** their governments

New Expressions	
anthropology /ˌænθrə'pɑːlədʒi/ *n.* 人类学	**hypothesis** /haɪ'pɑːθəsɪs/ *n.*（有少量事实依据但未被证实的）假说，假设
draw upon 利用	
linguistic /lɪŋ'gwɪstɪk/ *adj.* 语言学的	**consultant** /kən'sʌltənt/ *n.* 顾问
pluralistic /ˌplʊrə'lɪstɪk/ *adj.* 多元性的；多元化的	**rhetoric** /'retərɪk/ *n.* 华而不实的言语；花言巧语
attentive /ə'tentɪv/ *adj.* 注意的；专心的；留心的	**strengthen** /'streŋθn/ *v.* 加强；增强；巩固

---

① The text is adapted from the following sources: Society for Medical Anthropology. 2018. What is medical anthropology? *Society for Medical Anthropology*. Retrieved March 21, 2023, from Society for Medical Anthropology website.

Aronoff, M. J. 1998. Medical anthropology. *Encyclopedia Britannica*. Retrieved March 21, 2023, from Encyclopedia Britannica website.

 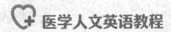

and **forestall** revolutionary **discontent**. In these countries—in **stark** contrast to countries with advanced economies—infectious diseases were the main cause of illness and death, and in many regions 50 percent or more of the infants born every year died before their fifth birthday. From 1945 through the 1960s, antibiotics were transforming the treatment of infectious diseases. Their use, combined with **immunization** of children, **sanitation**, and improved **nutrition**, was in the forefront of large-scale foreign aid programs.

The physicians who planned and directed health care projects at that time were almost immediately confronted with failure when townspeople **underutilized** their clinics, ignored instructions to boil water, or in other ways failed to comply with professional advice. Project workers were **convinced** that local cultural traditions formed a **superstitious** barrier to the rational behavior that they **advocated**. In this early period the anthropologists they consulted usually accepted their formulation of the problem, but they encouraged a degree of cultural relativism by suggesting ways that programs could acknowledge local customs and use traditional concepts to explain desirable new practices. This approach was illustrated in *Health, Culture, and Community*, a collection of case studies first presented at the Harvard School of Public Health. The volume became a basic text among teachers who in the 1960s were encouraged to **initiate** graduate programs in medical anthropology.

Shamanism[1] and other forms of **ritual curing** had been a major topic in anthropology from the beginning of the discipline, but the first studies of the whole **repertoire** of illness concepts and therapeutic practices available to members of a community began in the 1960s and 1970s. These years were a time of political **turmoil** in which anthropology was criticized as an **artifact** of European and American colonialism. Thus, students

New Expressions

forestall /fɔːrˈstɔːl/ v. 预先阻止；在（他人）之前行动；先发制人

discontent /ˌdɪskənˈtent/ n. 不满；不满足；不满足的缘由

stark /stɑːrk/ adj.（指区别）明显的，鲜明的

immunization /ˌɪmjunəˈzeɪʃn/ n. 免疫

sanitation /ˌsænɪˈteɪʃn/ n. 卫生设备；卫生设施体系

nutrition /nuˈtrɪʃn/ n. 营养；滋养；营养的补给

underutilize /ˌʌndərˈjuːtɪlaɪz/ v. 未充分使用

convince /kənˈvɪns/ v. 使确信；使相信；使信服

superstitious /ˌsuːpərˈstɪʃəs/ adj. 迷信的；有迷信观念的

advocate /ˈædvəkeɪt/ v. 拥护；支持；提倡

initiate /ɪˈnɪʃieɪt/ v. 开始；发起；创始

ritual curing 仪式疗法

repertoire /ˈrepərtwɑːr/ n.（某人的）全部才能，全部本领；（总称某人的）可表演项目

turmoil /ˈtɜːrmɔɪl/ n. 动乱；骚动；混乱；焦虑

artifact /ˈɑːrtɪfækt/ n. 人工制品；（尤指有历史或文化价值的）手工艺品

were **alert to** historical conflicts and injustice in the communities they studied, many of which were undergoing processes of **decolonization**. In addition, **the tradition-modernity dichotomy**[2], which then **dominated** research on cultural change, seemed to have little analytic value for understanding folk practitioners who were adding antibiotic injections to their repertoire of ritual curing and herbal remedies. Indeed, in their own society the rationality of modern Western medicine was challenged by scholars who **faulted** its **epistemology**—in particular, its **positivist** separation of mind and body, its dehumanizing focus on body parts, malfunctions, and **lesions**, and its treatment of pregnancy, birthing, and homosexuality as **pathological** rather than normal conditions.

The consulting work that originally focused anthropological attention on issues of health care was often **ad hoc**, but it did draw upon previous **functionalist studies of acculturation**[3]. The second generation of scholars, who brought medical anthropology to maturity as a special field of research, considered functionalism to be a **tautological** and politically conservative set of theories. Their work, which began to be published in the 1970s, was inspired by socialist thought, **French structuralism**[4], **dynamic** theories in **psychological anthropology**[5], and interpretive studies of **cultural symbolism**[6].

Americans took the lead in developing medical anthropology as a distinctive field of scholarship and practical work, but European scholars and practitioners have also founded specialist societies, journals, and monograph series. As the field expanded, subspecialties focused on issues, such as infectious diseases, aging, and nutrition emerged.

New Expressions	
be alert to 对……保持警惕	**positivist** /ˈpɑːzətɪvɪst/ *adj.* 实证主义的
decolonization /diːˌkɑːlənəˈzeɪʃn/ *n.* 非殖民（地）化	**lesion** /ˈliːʒn/ *n.* （因伤病导致皮肤或器官的）损伤，损害
dichotomy /daɪˈkɑːtəmi/ *n.* 一分为二；二分法	**pathological** /ˌpæθəˈlɑːdʒɪkl/ *adj.* 病态的；与疾病有关的
dominate /ˈdɑːmɪneɪt/ *v.* 支配；控制；左右；影响	**ad hoc** 临时安排的
fault /fɔːlt/ *v.* 发现错误；找出缺点	**tautological** /ˌtɔːtəˈlɑːdʒɪkl/ *adj.* 同义反复的
epistemology /ɪˌpɪstəˈmɑːlədʒi/ *n.* 认识论	**dynamic** /daɪˈnæmɪk/ *adj.* 动态的；发展变化的

1. **Shamanism**: 萨满教。萨满教是原始宗教的一种。萨满教信仰中的萨满被认为是掌握神秘知识、有能力进入"人神"状态的人，有着预言、治疗、与属灵世界沟通，以及旅行到属灵世界的能力。Historically, it is often associated with indigenous and tribal societies, and involves belief that shamans, with a connection to the otherworld, have the power to heal the sick, communicate with spirits, and escort souls of the dead to the afterlife.

2. **the tradition-modernity dichotomy**: 传统与现代二分法。它形成于 20 世纪五六十年代。其中，现代化被认为是典型的西方过程，非西方社会只有摒弃自己的传统文化才能接受现代化。但这一理论受到了很多批评与质疑。许多理论家强调，社会系统并非简单的二元对立，尽管在现代化的过程中经济和政治发生了变化，但传统价值仍然存在。In the social sciences, tradition is often contrasted with modernity, particularly in terms of whole societies. This dichotomy is generally associated with a linear model of social change, in which societies progress from being traditional to being modern. Tradition-oriented societies have been characterized as valuing filial piety, harmony and group welfare, stability, and interdependence, while a society exhibiting modernity would value individualism (with free will and choice), mobility, and progress.

3. **functionalist studies of acculturation**: 功能主义视角下的文化适应研究。根据功能主义理论，文化是一种集成的信仰、价值观、规范和实践系统，具有重要的社会功能，如促进社会凝聚力、维持社会秩序，并为个人提供意义和目的感。Functionalist studies of acculturation emphasize the importance of cultural exchange and adaptation in promoting social integration and stability, and suggest that cultural diversity can be a positive force for social progress and development.

4. **French structuralism**: 法国结构主义学派。该学派兴起于 20 世纪 60 年代，是俄国形式主义和布拉格学派的逻辑延伸，主要代表人物有列维－斯特劳斯、热奈特、戈德曼、阿尔都塞、格雷马斯、拉康等。French structuralism rose to prominence in the 1960s. Representative scholars in this field include Claude Lévi-Strauss, Gérard Genette, Lucien Gaudin, Louis Althusser, Algirdas Greimas, Jacques Lacan, etc.

5. **psychological anthropology**: 心理人类学。美籍华裔人类学家许烺光是该学科的奠基者。心理人类学是使用人类学概念和方法研究心理学课题的学科，可以被视为研究社会的一种视角，同时也是人类学的一个跨学科子领域。心理人类学倾向于关注人类在特定文化群体中的发展和适应方式如何塑造人类的认知、情感、感知、动机和心理。心理人类学存在多种不同的研究流派，如精神分析人类学、认知人类学、精神病人类学等。Psychological anthropology is the study of psychological topics using anthropological concepts and methods. Among the areas of interest are personal identity, selfhood, subjectivity, memory, consciousness, emotion, motivation, cognition, madness, and mental health. Francis L. K. Hsu has made foundational contributions to the development of psychological anthropology.

6. **cultural symbolism:** 文化象征主义。象征主义是 19 世纪末在法国及西方几个国家出现的一种艺术思潮，与现实主义相对立。文化象征主义是指使用物品、图像或行动来代表深深根植于特定文化中的抽象思想或价值观。这些象征符号可以用来表达广泛的概念：从宗教信仰和政治意识形态到社会规范和个人身份。In many cultures, symbolism plays a crucial role in shaping social practices and attitudes, as well as in communicating important cultural messages across generations. Cultural symbols can also be used to express collective identity and group belonging, as they often represent shared values and beliefs that are integral to a particular cultural group.

Post-reading Activities

I Speaking Practice: Group Discussion

Directions: *Please discuss the following questions in small groups. After your discussion, please share your opinions with the whole class.*

1. Based on your reading, what have you learned about medical anthropology?

2. What is the origin of medical anthropology? When and why are scholars specialized in anthropology invited to involve in projects in the health and medical context?

3. What were the problems and difficulties physicians faced when they planned and directed health care projects after World War Ⅱ? Were the problems and difficulties solved? If yes, in what ways?

II Speaking Practice: Oral Presentation

Directions: *From the text, it is known that both American and European scholars have founded specialist societies, journals, and monograph series on medical anthropology. Please search for the information on societies and international journals in relation to medical anthropology on the Internet. Then, please give an oral presentation to introduce at least one society or academic journal in this field. Your presentation should include the target, mission and features of the society or journal chosen.*

Part 2 Thematic Reading

Ethnomedicine[①]

Ethnomedicine is the area of anthropology that studies different societies' notions of health and illness, including how people think and how people act about well-being and healing. Medicine—like language, music and politics—is a subset of culture which is situated locally. Thus, we have British medicine, **Bavarian medicine, Massai medicine, Mayan medicine**[1], and so forth. Each society has its own medical style, or medical culture. Beliefs about the body and illness causation, together with societal norms concerning when, why, and who to seek for medical help comprise one's "culture of medicine", or ethnomedicine. Although related societies may share some ethnomedical beliefs, just as linguistic dialects and political circumstances even of close cultures may **diverge**, so may their medical views. It is safe to **assume** that there are as many unique medical perspectives, or ethnomedicines, as there are cultures and subcultures. Every society's medicine (the West included) and every type and branch of medicine is "**potential fodder**" for ethnomedical study.

The term "ethnomedicine" appears in academic literature with somewhat different meanings. In the American anthropological literature, the "medicine" in "ethnomedicine" usually refers to knowledge and ideas about health and health care. In European and biological literature, the "medicine" tends to refer to medication or treatment practices. In fact, the English word "medicine" is not a precise term, but a general one that, in any dictionary, has several related definitions dealing with knowledge about several areas

New Expressions	
ethnomedicine /ˌeθnoʊˈmedɪsn/ *n.* 民族医学	**potential** /pəˈtenʃl/ *adj.* 潜在的；可能的
diverge /daɪˈvɜːrdʒ/ *v.*（意见、观点等）分歧，相异	**fodder** /ˈfɑːdər/ *n.*（人或东西）只能是……的料；素材
assume /əˈsuːm/ *v.* 假定；假设；认为	

① The text is adapted from the following source: Quinlan, M. B. 2011. Ethnomedicine. In M. Singer & P. I. Erickson (Eds.), *A Companion to Medical Anthropology*. Hoboken: Wiley-Blackwell, 381–403.

 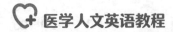

including health, the body, illness causes, prevention, diagnosis and treatment. Just as these types of knowledge are all "medicine" in the English-speaking world, so they are all ethnomedicine when describing the medicine of any particular culture.

As is typical for fields with the **"ethno" prefix**[2], ethnomedicine seeks out primarily an **"emic" anthropological view**[3], i.e. the perspective of a member of the culture being studied. Emic views are not easy for an outsider to come by because they reflect developmental experience within a particular local framework. Strangely enough, it often takes an outside vantage to clarify an emic system (much as an outside psychotherapist can help untangle patterns from the **"noise"**[4] in a patient's social history). A foreign researcher who meets medical issues with an outsider's or **"etic" perspective**[5] can recognize and inquire about cognitive and behavioral models that a native of the culture may take for granted or not notice. Medical anthropologists usually learn emic health views through fieldwork among people from a particular culture.

Ethnomedicine has two basic goals. First, it examines the health related theories and knowledge that people inherit and learn by living in a culture. This information forms the base of a culture's medical common sense, or medical logic that people use to explain and treat their illnesses. Ethnomedicine's other goal is medical translation. We seek not only to understand the medical thinking of one group, but to compare ideas cross-culturally for regional and global understanding. Translation of ethnomedical knowledge is applicable to improve health care delivery for the group studied, or to inform alternative health practices for Western and other societies.

Ethnomedicine is a touchy subject for many. Examination of varied medical practices attracts some people and repulses others. Anthropological translation of the foreign emic beliefs of some culture can make them understandable etically[6] to people from other cultures. For the Westerners, the etic perspective is almost always the bioscientific one.

New Expressions	
come by 来到；得到；理解	inherit /ɪn'herɪt/ v. 经遗传获得（品质、身体特征等）
vantage /'væntɪdʒ/ n. 优势；有利地位	
psychotherapist /ˌsaɪkoʊ'θerəpɪst/ n. 心理治疗医师；精神治疗医生	alternative /ɔːl'tɜːnətɪv/ adj. 可供替代的；非传统的
untangle /ˌʌn'tæŋgl/ v. 整理；厘清	repulse /rɪ'pʌls/ v. 使厌恶；使反感
inquire /ɪn'kwaɪər/ v. 询问；打听	

Browner et al. propose a way to "combine the emic perspective of ethnomedicine with the etic measures of bioscience". Following their methods, the researcher identifies the health problem and how it is **conceivably** healed according to the locals, objectively **assesses** the remedy's ability to produce the **emically**[7] desired effect, and identifies the areas of **convergence** and divergence between the emic and the etic assessments. For example, these authors suggest that **Aztecs**[8] **envisioned** some headaches as the result of a build-up of blood in the head. Many Aztec headache medicines produced nasal bleeding, which was presumably thought to release the feeling of pressure **allegedly** caused by the excess blood in the head. These medicines were effective in Aztec terms because they achieved the desired result (i.e. a bloody nose). From the etic perspective, Aztec medications have chemical properties capable of causing nosebleeds, though most remain scientifically **undemonstrated** as headache remedies.

Anthropology's tradition of moving from etic to emic inquiry perhaps **obstructed** the study of Western medical culture, particularly biomedicine, even though it is one of the world's many ethnomedicines. Only recently, in the late 20th century, have medical anthropologists, informed by other medical systems' perspectives, begun to study and constructively critique biomedicine as an ethnomedical system. Ethnomedical research nevertheless **persists** largely among foreign, minority, and **underserved** populations.

Knowledge of ethnomedical translation has become increasingly relevant for public health because it identifies beliefs and practices among the foreign, minority, and underserved. As mentioned, people tend to be **ethnocentric** about their medicine—they hold dearly to their own medical traditions. Globalization and the resulting increase in cultural contact leads to medical **incongruences**. Differences between groups' medical thinking become problematic when people from small-scale cultures migrate

New Expressions	
conceivably /kən'siːvəbli/ *adv.* 可想象地；可信地	**obstruct** /əb'strʌkt/ *v.* （故意）妨碍，阻挠，阻碍
assess /ə'ses/ *v.* 评估，评定（性质、质量）	**persist** /pər'sɪst/ *v.* 维持；保持；持续存在
convergence /kən'vɜːrdʒəns/ *n.* （思想、政策、目标等）十分相似，相同	**underserved** /ˌʌndər'sɜːrvd/ *adj.* 服务不周到的；服务水平低下的
envision /ɪn'vɪʒn/ *v.* 想象；设想；展望	**ethnocentric** /ˌeθnoʊ'sentrɪk/ *adj.* 种族（或民族）中心主义的；种族（或民族）优越感的
allegedly /ə'ledʒɪdli/ *adv.* 据说；据称	
undemonstrated /ˌʌn'demənstreɪtɪd/ *adj.* 未经证实的	**incongruence** /ɪn'kɑːŋgruəns/ *n.* 不一致；不协调

to developed areas where biomedicine dominates, illnesses spread to societies that have not experienced the illness before, and Western medicine **makes inroads to** areas of the globe in which biomedical traditions are new, foreign, and in some cases **suspect**. Understanding ethnomedical beliefs allows researchers to become medical **mediators**.

New Expressions	
make inroads to 侵入	**mediator** /'miːdieɪtər/ *n.* 调停者；斡旋者；解决纷争的人（或机构）
suspect /'sʌspekt/ *adj.* 不可信的；靠不住的	

Notes

1. **Bavarian medicine, Massai medicine, Mayan medicine:** 巴伐利亚医学、马赛医学、玛雅医学。巴伐利亚，全称巴伐利亚自由州，位于德国南部，是德国面积最大的联邦州。巴伐利亚医学指的是巴伐利亚人的传统治疗方法和健康信仰体系。马赛医学指的是马赛人的传统治疗方法和信仰。马赛人是一个半游牧民族，居住在东非肯尼亚和坦桑尼亚的部分地区。马赛人使用传统的草药疗法及精神和仪式等方法来促进健康和治疗疾病，历史悠久。马赛人的医学理念是：疾病是因人的身体、社会和精神方面的平衡被破坏而引起的。玛雅医学是指玛雅人的传统治疗方法和信仰。玛雅医学基于对健康和疾病的整体理解，承认一个人的身体、情感和精神方面的相互联系。传统的玛雅治疗师使用自然疗法、精神实践和仪式的组合来治疗疾病和促进愈合。玛雅医学还强调与自然界保持和谐关系的重要性，许多传统的治疗方法都与自然环境的节奏和周期紧密相连。These terms refer to traditional treatment approaches and beliefs in medicine adopted by the Bavarian, Massai, and Mayan.

2. **"ethno" prefix:** "民族" 前缀。ethno 意为 "民族""人种"。该词缀在人文社科领域较为常用，在人类学领域常见于 ethnography 一词。ethnography 可被译为 "民族志""人种志""人种学"，是指对人类特定社会开展的描述性研究范式、项目或过程。The prefix could be used in words, such as ethnography, which refers to a description of a people and/or their culture. Ethnography is a typical qualitative research method and process in social sciences.

3. **"emic" anthropological view:** 主位人类学观点。它是指内部人人类学视角与观念。emic 意为 "位的""着位的"，其在人文社科领域的常见搭配有 emic approach，意为 "主位研究""主位取向""主位途径"。It refers to the anthropological view which obtains viewpoints from within the social group and from the perspective of the subject.

4. the "noise": 杂音，不太相关的细节。这里指混杂在言语陈述中、对于了解病人的病史和情况表面上不起作用或不相关的信息。Noise here should be understood figuratively. It refers to the details that are irrelevant to the understanding of patients' history and situation.

5. "etic" perspective: 客位视角。它是指外部人视角。etic 意为"（对特定语言和文化的描述）非位的""素的"。Etic perspective means to obtain the viewpoints from outside the social group and from the perspective of the observer.

6. etically: 客位取向地，外部人视角地。这是形容词 etic 的副词形式。As the adverb of "etic", etically means "from the outsider's perspective".

7. emically: 主位取向地，内部人视角地。这是形容词 emic 的副词形式。As the adverb of "emic", emically means "from the insider's perspective".

8. Aztecs: 阿兹特克人。这是北美洲南部墨西哥人数最多的一支印第安人，其中心在墨西哥的特诺奇，故又被称为墨西哥人或特诺奇人。According to Aztec tradition, their people originated somewhere in the northwestern region of Mexico.

Post-reading Activities

I Language Building-up

Task 1 Extensive Vocabulary Enlargement

Directions: *The following words are taken from the text. Please follow the three-step learning in this part and build up your own Extensive Vocabulary Chart.*

Step 1. Read through the words and underline them in the text. Circle the ones that are particularly new to you. Look up the words in the dictionary and put the equivalent Chinese translation in the chart below.

Step 2. While you go back to the text, please feel free to put any other words into the blanks provided in the extra lines in the chart.

Extensive Vocabulary Chart				
ethnomedicine	assume	fodder	psychotherapist	untangle

Extensive Vocabulary Chart				
alternative	conceivably	assess	allegedly	undemonstrated
obstruct	persist	underserved	ethnocentric	incongruence

Step 3. Please group the above words based on their parts of speech and meanings.

Nouns	
Verbs	
Adjectives	
Adverbs and Prepositions	
Medical Terminology	
Terminology in Other Fields	

Task 2   Intensive Vocabulary Enhancement

Directions: *The following 10 words are chosen from the text. They will form the intensive vocabulary in this unit. For intensive vocabulary, you are supposed to be able to explain them in English and use them in sentence and discourse constructions.*

Step 1. Please read through the words and be familiar with their Chinese and English definitions. Recall where and how they are used in the text.

Intensive Vocabulary Chart				
No.	Word	Translation	Definition	Status
1	diverge	（意见、观点等）分歧；相异	v. (of opinions, views, etc.) to be different	☆ ☆ ☆ ☆ ☆
2	vantage	优势；有利地位	n. the advantage or superiority in a contest; a position or an opportunity likely to give superiority	☆ ☆ ☆ ☆ ☆
3	inquire	询问；打听	v. to ask sb. for some information	☆ ☆ ☆ ☆ ☆
4	inherit	经遗传获得（品质、身体特征等）	v. to have qualities, physical features, etc. that are similar to those of sb.'s parents, grandparents, etc.	☆ ☆ ☆ ☆ ☆
5	repulse	使厌恶；使反感	v. to make sb. feel disgust or strong dislike	☆ ☆ ☆ ☆ ☆
6	convergence	（思想、政策、目标等）十分相似，相同	n. ideas, policies, aims, etc. that become very similar or the same	☆ ☆ ☆ ☆ ☆
7	envision	想象；设想；展望	v. to imagine what a situation will be like in the future, especially a situation sb. intends to work towards	☆ ☆ ☆ ☆ ☆
8	persist	维持；保持；持续存在	v. to continue to exist	☆ ☆ ☆ ☆ ☆
9	suspect	不可信的；靠不住的	adj. that may be false and that cannot be relied on	☆ ☆ ☆ ☆ ☆
10	mediator	调停者；斡旋者；解决纷争的人（或机构）	n. a person or an organization that tries to get agreement between people or groups who disagree with each other	☆ ☆ ☆ ☆ ☆

Step 2. Please tick the status for each word based on your own situation. If one word is very new or difficult for you, please tick five stars. Likewise, if one word is comparatively easy for you and you don't have to spend too much time on reading and learning it, then tick one star. The number of stars represents the difficulty of commanding a word in your eyes.

Step 3. Please complete the following 10 sentences by choosing appropriate words from the Intensive Vocabulary Chart. Please change the forms of the words where necessary.

1. It's a fascinating _____ point from which to view the city.

   这是观察这座城市的一个有利角度。

2. Who will act as _____ in the dispute?

   谁在争端中充当调解人？

3. Opinions _____ greatly on this issue.

   在这个问题上意见分歧很大。

4. Some of the evidence they produced was highly _____

   他们出示的证据中有些相当成问题。

5. They _____ an equal society, free of poverty and disease.

   他们向往一个没有贫穷和疾病的平等社会。

6. I was _____ by the horrible smell.

   这种可怕的气味让我恶心。

7. There is a(n) _____ between capitalist firms and cooperatives in terms of business strategy.

   资本主义公司和合作企业在经营战略方面趋于一致。

8. The police are _____ into the murder case.

   警察正在调查这起谋杀案。

9. He has _____ his mother's patience.

   他的耐心遗传自其母亲。

10. If the symptoms _____, you should consult your doctor.

    如果症状持续不退，你就得去看医生。

Task 3   Expressions and Sentences

Directions: *The following sentences are taken from the text. In each sentence, there is one phrase being underlined. Please refer to the dictionary and write down the explanation of the phrase in the line entitled "Meaning Exploration". After that, please make a sentence with it. Write the sentence in the line entitled "Sentence Making".*

Sentence 1

Original Sentence	Emic views are not easy for an outsider to come by because they reflect developmental experience within a particular local framework.
Meaning Exploration	come by:

Sentence Making	

Sentence 2

Original Sentence	This information <u>forms the base of</u> a culture's medical common sense, or medical logic that people use to explain and treat their illnesses.
Meaning Exploration	*form the base of*:
Sentence Making	

Sentence 3

Original Sentence	Translation of ethnomedical knowledge <u>is applicable to</u> improve health care delivery for the group studied, or to inform alternative health practices for Western and other societies.
Meaning Exploration	*be applicable to*:
Sentence Making	

Sentence 4

Original Sentence	From the etic perspective, Aztec medications have chemical properties <u>capable of</u> causing nosebleeds, though most remain scientifically undemonstrated as headache remedies.
Meaning Exploration	*capable of*:
Sentence Making	

Sentence 5

Original Sentence	Globalization and the resulting increase in cultural contact <u>leads to</u> medical incongruences.
Meaning Exploration	*lead to*:

Sentence Making	

ⅠⅠ Critical Reading and Thinking

Task 1 Overview and Comprehension

Directions: *While reading an article, it is a good habit to take down some reading notes. Reading notes usually include the main idea and key information provided in the article. Please read through the text and provide the missing information in the following Reading Notes.*

Reading Notes	
Definition of Ethnomedicine	
Two Goals for Ethnomedicine	
The Value of Ethnomedical Translation	

Task 2 Reflection and Discussion

Directions: *After reading, please reflect on the theme of the text. Work in groups and share your opinions on the following questions with other group members.*

1. At the beginning of the text, the author said "Medicine—like language, music and politics—is a subset of culture which is situated locally." Can you compare medicine to language, music and politics? Please talk about your understanding of this statement with examples to illustrate your ideas.

2. Based on your reading, what should medical researchers and practitioners do to translate ethnomedical knowledge to improve the quality of health care?

3. In what circumstances will the differences between groups' medical thinking become problematic? What are the potential problems?

4. What are the opportunities and challenges traditional Chinese medicine face when modern Western medicine becomes prevalent in China?

医学人文英语教程

Part 3 Extended Reading

Culture and Health[①]

Have you ever felt when you went to the doctor that your problem wasn't understood or that your treatment was not relevant to your health problem? Cultural differences between physicians and their diverse clients make cross-cultural misunderstandings inevitable. Culture affects patients' and providers' **perceptions** of health conditions and appropriate treatments. Culture also affects behaviors that **expose** us **to** disease and the reasons **prompting** us to seek care, how we describe our symptoms, and our **compliance** with treatments. This makes culture central to diagnosis and an important issue for all of the health professions.

Patients and providers need knowledge of the relationships of culture to health because culture is the foundation of everyone's health concerns and practices. Improving health care requires attention to cultural influences on health concerns, conditions, beliefs, and practices. People's health occurs within cultural systems that are concerned with broader issues of well-being than addressed by physicians' concerns with disease and injury; we are also concerned with psychological, social, emotional, mental, and spiritual well-being. As biomedicine turns from a disease-focused approach to concepts with health and well-being, cultural perspectives and cultural competency emerge as central frameworks for improving care.

Medical anthropology is the primary discipline addressing the **interfaces** of medicine, culture, and health behavior and incorporating cultural perspectives into

New Expressions	
perception /pər'sepʃn/ *n.* 知觉；感知；洞察力；见解	**compliance** /kəm'plaɪəns/ *n.* 服从；顺从；遵从
expose... to　使面临，使遭受（危险或不快）	**interface** /'ɪntərfeɪs/ *n.* （两学科、体系等的）接合点，边缘区域
prompt /prɑːmpt/ *v.* 促使；导致；激起	

① The text is adapted from the following source: Winkelman, M. 2008. Applied medical anthropology and health care. In M. Winkelman (Ed.), *Culture and Health: Applying Medical Anthropology* (1st ed.). San Francisco: Jossey-Bass, 1–25.

clinical settings and public health programs. Health professionals need knowledge of culture and cross-cultural relationship skills because health services are more effective when responsive to cultural needs. Cross-cultural skills also are important in relationships among providers of different cultures when, for example, African American and Filipino nurses interact with each other or with Anglo, Hispanic, or Hindu physicians. A knowledge of culture is also necessary for work in community settings, such as collaborating with diverse groups and organizations to develop culturally relevant public health programs. Health care providers and patients are more effective in managing their health and care with cultural awareness and the ability to manage the numerous factors that affect well-being.

What do health professionals need to know about the effects of culture on health? They all need systematic ways of studying cultural effects on health and developing cultural competence. Cultural **responsiveness** is necessary for providers, researchers, and educators if they are to be effective in relating to others across the barriers of cultural differences. The cultural perspectives of medical anthropology are **essential** for providing competent care, effective community health programs, and patient education. For biomedicine to be effective, providers need to know whether a patient views the physician as believable and **trustworthy**, the diagnosis as acceptable, the symptoms as problematic, and the treatment as accessible and effective.

The concept of culture is fundamental to understanding health and medicine because personal health behaviors and professional practices of medicine are deeply influenced by culture. Culture involves the learned patterns of shared group behaviors. These learned shared behaviors are the framework for understanding and explaining all human behavior. This includes health behaviors, particularly intergroup differences in health behaviors and beliefs. Culture is a principal determinant of health conditions, particularly in exposing us to or protecting us from diseases through structuring our interactions with the physical and social environments. Culture also defines the kinds of health problems that exist and the resources for responding to health concerns, defining our perceptions, and producing the resources for responding to them.

New Expressions

responsiveness /rɪ'spɑːnsɪvnəs/ *n.* 敏感度；响应性

essential /ɪ'senʃl/ *adj.* 必不可少的；完全必要的；极其重要的

trustworthy /'trʌstwɜːrði/ *adj.* 值得信赖的

Cultural knowledge is also essential for addressing public health mandates to assess communities' health needs, develop appropriate health policies and programs, and ensure adequate and culturally competent health services. The health needs of communities vary widely, requiring an understanding of each community's perceptions of health and illness to develop appropriate services. Public health initiatives require knowledge of culture to change the behaviors and lifestyles associated with an increased incidence of disease. Addressing the effects of culture on health is an important issue for everyone, not just physicians, because disease in any group impacts society as a whole. According to Durch, Bailey, and Stoto, "Improving health is a shared responsibility of health care providers, public health officials, and a variety of other actors in the community." This requires people with an ability to engage communities in a culturally appropriate manner and understanding of their cultural systems, health beliefs, and practices.

Health service professionals face common concerns in addressing how culture affects relations with individual clients and how their well-being is produced in interaction with many aspects of the environment. Effectively addressing these concerns requires cultural competence, which includes both individual and organizational capacities, behaviors, attitudes, and policies that effectively address cultural differences through the use of cultural knowledge and intercultural skills. Cultural competence involves the ability to address a range of cultural factors.

Knowledge of cultural systems and organizational culture is part of the ability to address clients' problems by recognizing economic, political, and other social factors that have effects on well-being and health behaviors. Effectively adapting to others' health behaviors requires knowledge of both their cultural influences and the effects of the provider's culture. These differences can produce conflicts that impede effective cross-cultural relations and clinical communication. Cultural knowledge and intercultural skills together can help overcome these barriers through an accommodation to the cross-cultural realities of clinical care and public health.

New Expressions

mandate /'mændeɪt/ *n.* （政府或组织等经选举而获得的）授权

initiative /ɪ'nɪʃətɪv/ *n.* 倡议；新方案

impact /ɪm'pækt/ *v.* （对某事物）有影响，有作用

impede /ɪm'piːd/ *v.* 阻碍；阻止

accommodation /ə,kɑːmə'deɪʃn/ *n.* 和解；调解；调和

Cultural competence levels range from **destructiveness (ethnocentrism)**, incapacity, and blindness through varying degrees of skill represented in the concepts of cultural awareness, sensitivity, responsiveness, competence, and proficiency. Awareness of cultural differences may be followed by sensitivity in response to them. Competence involves the capability to deal effectively with cultural differences. Proficiency involves the ability to transfer this knowledge and these skills to others. Cultural awareness and sensitivity assist in adapting to other cultures through a knowledge of specific cultural information and the ability to provide culturally responsive care by addressing general barriers to effective cross-cultural relations. The ability to deal with cultural differences begins with overcoming ethnocentrism and developing an awareness of other cultures that leads to an understanding of the more sophisticated skills necessary to adapt effectively to cultural differences and intercultural processes.

What's more, cultural competence requires personal cultural awareness and an understanding of one's own professional culture and its unconscious **assumptions**, values, and motivations that affect patient relations. Learning about the effects of one's culture on health expectations and the medical encounter provides the basis for understanding intercultural conflicts in provider-patient relations and enhancing patient care by providing caregivers and consumers greater knowledge of one another.

New Expressions	
destructiveness /dɪˈstrʌktɪvnəs/ *n.* 破坏性	**assumption** /əˈsʌmpʃn/ *n.* 假设；假定
ethnocentrism /ˌeθnoʊˈsentrɪzəm/ *n.* 民族中心 主义	

Post-reading Activities

I Speaking Practice: Role Play

Directions: *Please work in pairs. Imagine one of you is a doctor in traditional Chinese medicine, and the other is a patient from a Western country who travels to China. The patient suffers from a serious cold, which causes coughing, nose running,*

医学人文英语教程

and a headache. Please design a conversation between the doctor and the patient during which the doctor prescribes some mild traditional Chinese medicine and advises the patient to drink more water and take more rest, while the patient insists on asking the doctor to prescribe some Western medications to cure the cold as he/she usually does back in his/her country. Be sure to present the importance of recognizing cultural knowledge and adopting intercultural skills in doctor-patient communication. Please take turns to be the doctor and the patient.

II Reflective Writing Practice: Short Essay

Directions: *Culture is the foundation of everyone's health concerns and practices, and the cultural competence of health professionals can eventually affect treatment outcomes. Please think about the definition, importance, and ways of improving cultural competence among health professionals, and write a reflective essay entitled "Cultural Competence in Health Professions". Please use some concrete examples to illustrate your ideas. The word limit is suggested to be 150–200 words.*

Unit 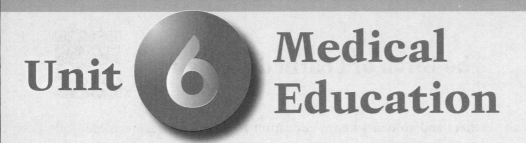 Medical Education

> *To study the phenomena of disease without books is to sail an uncharted sea, while to study books without patients is not to go to sea at all.*
>
> —William Osler

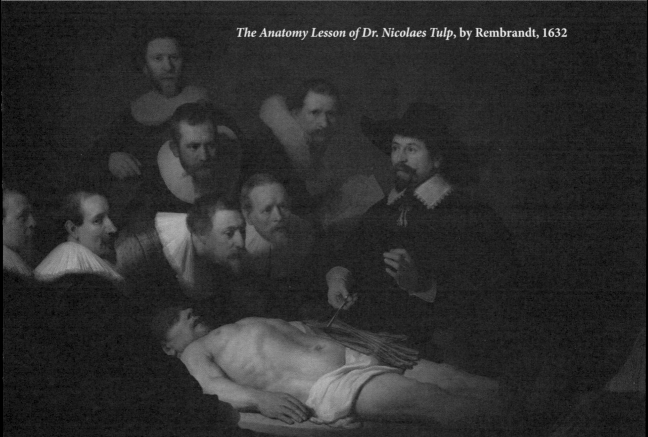

The Anatomy Lesson of Dr. Nicolaes Tulp, by Rembrandt, 1632

Part 1 Academic Horizon

The Birth of Learned Medicine[①]

As all teachers and students know, education is a difficult business. Medical education is especially difficult because people's lives are **at stake** and because the **acquisition** of scientific and clinical knowledge is such a demanding process. The history of medical education is characterized by constant **pedagogical** tensions. This text sketches the stages of development of medical education in **antiquity** in the context of Western Europe and the United States.

Traditionally, formally trained medical students came from **privileged** family backgrounds. In ancient India, for example, the ***Charaka Samhita***[1], an Ayurvedic Sanskrit text from the 3rd century BCE, advised teachers to seek students who were associated with or came from a family of doctors. Teachers **urged** their students "to be **chaste** and **temperate**, to speak the truth, to obey... in all things and to wear a beard". In addition to a robust beard, discipline and integrity were essential. In ancient Egypt, medical students often lived under the strict supervision and direction of their teachers. One **treatise** demonstrates that some student **recreational** habits seem unaffected by history.

Before the 5th century BCE, Greek medicine was characterized by two kinds of

New Expressions	
at stake 有风险	优待的
acquisition /ˌækwɪˈzɪʃn/ *n.*（知识、技能等的）获得，得到	**urge** /ɜːrdʒ/ *v.* 敦促；催促；力劝
pedagogical /ˌpedəˈɡɑːdʒɪkl/ *adj.* 教学法的	**chaste** /tʃeɪst/ *adj.* 贞洁的；忠贞的
antiquity /ænˈtɪkwəti/ *n.* 古代（尤指古希腊和古罗马时期）	**temperate** /ˈtempərət/ *adj.* 温和的；心平气和的；自我克制的
privileged /ˈprɪvəlɪdʒd/ *adj.* 有特权的；受特别	**treatise** /ˈtriːtɪs/ *n.*（专题）论文
	recreational /ˌrekriˈeɪʃənl/ *adj.* 娱乐的；消遣的

① The text is adapted from the following source: Cole, R. T. et al. 2015. *Medical Humanities: An Introduction*. New York: Cambridge University Press.

 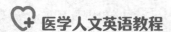

knowledge: secular **traumatology** (the care of wounds, injuries, and broken bones) and supernatural **revelation** (the wisdom of the gods). In the first case, a **resident** or wandering craftsman **imparted** knowledge orally and by practice, usually from father to son. The second kind of practitioner—the priest as physician—imparted religious wisdom to his **initiates**. This situation was altered when the Hippocratics (c. 400 BCE) separated medical from religious explanation and produced the first secular medical texts. Despite the influence of the *Hippocratic Corpus*, its pedagogical value was often **called into question**. Aristotle (384—322 BCE), whose father was a physician, commented on the **perennial** tension between textual and clinical learning: "Clearly you do not become a physician by books... the writers of books try to describe... the general... methods of **therapeutics**. That would be useful for the skilled man but the untrained one gains no use from it."

In 323 BCE, teachers at the world's largest and most famous library—the "Musaeum" at Alexandria—invented new educational formats that later became known as lectures and seminars. In medicine, competing **sects** produced rival educational forms. Herophilus of Chalcedon (335—280 BCE) undertook the first formal **dissections** of human bodies, which in turn became part of the education of physicians. In contrast, the **empiricists** claimed that the knowledge of internal human processes could only be learned from the experience of caring for patients. After Alexandria passed into the Roman rule in 80 BCE, Roman hostility to Greek philosophy and science led to a shorter and less theoretical style of education. Roman physician Thessalus (c. 70—95 AD), who popularized the study of medicine, claimed that he could transform a student into a physician in six months.

During the Hellenistic Period (326 BCE—146 AD) an **amalgam** of Greek, Jewish, and Egyptian cultures yielded more open social norms and popular forms of medical

New Expressions	
traumatology /ˌtrɑːmə'tɑlədʒi/ *n.* 创伤学；外伤学	**call into question** 对……表示怀疑
revelation /ˌrevə'leɪʃn/ *n.* （上帝的）启示	**perennial** /pə'reniəl/ *adj.* 长久的；持续的；反复出现的
resident /'rezɪdənt/ *n.* （美国的）高级专科住院实习医生	**therapeutics** /ˌθerə'pjuːtɪks/ *n.* 治疗学
impart /ɪm'pɑːrt/ *v.* 通知；透露；传授	**sect** /sekt/ *n.* 派别；宗派
	dissection /daɪ'sekʃn/ *n.* 分析
initiate /ɪ'nɪʃiət/ *n.* 新加入某组织（或机构、宗教）的人；新入会的人	**empiricist** /ɪm'pɪrɪsɪst/ *n.* 经验主义者
	amalgam /ə'mælgəm/ *n.* 混合物；综合体

knowledge. Some writers called for medical knowledge to be taught as part of general public education, leading to occasional public lectures and advice for laymen in need of sudden medical assistance. The term "*iatrine*[2]" (meaning a woman physician) signified authority and jurisdiction that occasionally went beyond the traditional expectations of women as midwives. Male physician Heracleides of Taras, for example, wrote to a woman physician, Antiochis, addressing her as a colleague and providing clinical advice. In general, however, the ideal physician was expected to be a healthy, courteous male from a lofty social position.

In the tradition of learned medicine, Galen's (c. 131—c. 201 BCE) ambiguous attitude toward books exemplified the perennial tension between textual and clinical education. On the one hand, he argued that books undermined the importance of seeing with one's own eyes. On the other hand, Galen wrote up to 600 treatises and employed scribes to write down his words. Indeed, the works of Hippocrates (c. 460—370 BCE) and Galen came to be regarded as infallible sources of medical knowledge—which both fostered and limited the growth of education and research—for more than 1,500 years.

After the fall of the Roman Empire in the 5th century, the urban life of antiquity was replaced by a medieval countryside that was dotted with castles and cathedrals. Learned medical practice and teaching virtually disappeared. Although some manuscripts were preserved and studied in European cathedrals and monasteries, the center of medical knowledge and learning shifted to the East. During the 8th century, scores of Greek texts were translated into Arabic, including Hippocrates' major texts and 129 of Galen's works. The *Firdaws al-hikma*, a medical compendium by Ali ibn Sahl Rabban al-Tabari (c. 838—870 AD), contained Arab translations of not only Hippocrates, Galen, and other

New Expressions	
signify /'sɪɡnɪfaɪ/ v. 表示；说明；预示	员，抄书吏
courteous /'kɜːrtiəs/ adj. 有礼貌的；客气的；（尤指）恭敬的，谦恭的	infallible /ɪn'fæləbl/ adj. 永无过失的；一贯正确的
lofty /'lɑːfti/ adj. 崇高的；高尚的	dot /dɑːt/ v. 星罗棋布于；遍布
ambiguous /æm'bɪɡjuəs/ adj. 不明确的	cathedral /kə'θiːdrəl/ n. 主教座堂；教区总教堂
exemplify /ɪɡ'zemplɪfaɪ/ v. 举例说明；例证；例示	manuscript /'mænjuskrɪpt/ n. （印刷术发明以前书籍或文献的）手写本，手抄本
undermine /ˌʌndər'maɪn/ v. 逐渐削弱（信心、权威等）；使逐步减少效力	score /skɔːr/ n. 大量，很多（常用复数）
scribe /skraɪb/ n. （印刷术发明之前的）抄写	compendium /kəm'pendiəm/ n. （尤指书中某题材事实、图画及照片的）汇编，概要

Greek writers but also texts from the Persian and Indian traditions. Arabic scholars thus preserved classical Western medical knowledge that would otherwise have been lost and made their own contributions as well.

In a largely rural European society, very few people read at all, let alone medical texts, which were written in Latin, **scattered** among monasteries and a few cities, and hand-copied on **parchment** made from the skin of sheep and cattle. **Aspiring** medical students, however, were expected to possess knowledge of the classical liberal arts by the age of fifteen. From the 9th century, medical texts balanced classical philosophy with practical advice and observation. "From what signs do you diagnose **melancholia**?" asked one treatise. Answer:

> From a distaste for life and dislike of other people's company; from the sadness of the **countenance**, from the silence, suspicion, and irrational weeping of the patient...

This question-and-answer format implies the existence of a student-teacher relationship, although its nature and frequency cannot be documented. Medical texts often warned students against drunkenness, overeating, **consorting** with women of ill **repute**, or any activity that could damage one's mind.

Formal medical education in the west appeared with the founding of universities at Paris (1110), Bologna (1158), Oxford (1167), Montpellier (1181), Cambridge (1209), Padua (1222), and Naples (1224). Padua and Bologna offered the most advanced medical education and attracted students from across Europe. Like the other learned professions of law and theology, medicine **anchored** itself in textual analysis. By the end of the 12th century, medical education had become a process of learning set **doctrines** in unquestioned traditional texts. Learned physicians and church officials tended to **disparage** surgery, which was considered a "lower", less refined art. However, itinerant

New Expressions	
scatter /'skætər/ *v.* 撒；撒播	**consort** /kən'sɔːrt/ *v.* 厮混；鬼混
parchment /'pɑːrtʃmənt/ *n.* 羊皮纸	**repute** /rɪ'pjuːt/ *n.* 名誉；名声
aspiring /ə'spaɪərɪŋ/ *adj.* 有抱负的；有志向的	**anchor** /'æŋkər/ *v.* 使扎根；使基于
melancholia /ˌmelən'koʊliə/ *n.* 忧郁症	**doctrine** /'dɑːktrɪn/ *n.* 教义；主义；学说；信条
countenance /'kaʊntənəns/ *n.* 面容；脸色；面部表情	**disparage** /dɪ'spærɪdʒ/ *v.* 贬低；轻视

surgeons who practiced their **craft** daily were likely more skilled than those who taught from books and occasional practice.

New Expression
craft /kræft/ *n.* 技巧；技能；技艺

Notes

1. *Charaka Samhita:*《阇罗迦集》。这是古代吠陀医生查茹阿卡撰写的、论述详尽的梵语阿育吠陀医学书籍，受到了人们极大的尊崇。It is a Sanskrit text on Ayurveda (traditional Indian medicine) which is considered to be one of the two foundational Hindu texts of this field that have survived from ancient India.

2. *iatrine*: 女医生。iatro- 为希腊语词根，表示"医学""医师"之意。It is a word root in Greek. Its meaning is in relation to medicine and physicians.

Post-reading Activities

I **Speaking Practice: Group Discussion**

Directions: *Please discuss the following questions in small groups. After your discussion, please share your opinions with the whole class.*

1. What qualities must formally trained medical students possess in tradition?
2. What is known about Greek medicine before the 5th century BCE?
3. What are the contributions made by Arabic scholars to Western medical knowledge?
4. When and how did the center of medical knowledge and learning shift to the East?

II Speaking Practice: Oral Presentation

Directions: *According to the text, we know that since the very beginning of medical education, there have been concerns over the tension between textual education and clinical education. What is the relationship between textual education and clinical education in medical education nowadays? Please give an oral presentation to share your opinions on the actual and ideal relationship between them.*

Part 2 Thematic Reading

Competency-based Medical Education^①

Competency-based educational models are not new. In other fields, this is often called competency-based education and training (CBET), a term transformed to competency-based medical education (CBME) in medicine. What is CBET? As Sullivan notes: "In a traditional educational system, the unit of **progression** is time and it is teacher-centered. In a CBET system, the unit of progression is mastery of specific knowledge and skills and is learner-centered."

The earliest **conception** of competency-based training arose in the United States during the 1920s as educational reform became linked to industrial and business models of work that centered on clear specification of outcomes and the associated knowledge and skills needed. However, the more recent conception of CBET had much of its **genesis** in the teacher education reform movement of the 1960s. This interest was **spurred** by a U.S. Office of Education National Center for Education Research grant program. In 1968, 10 universities developed and implemented new teacher training models that focused on student achievement. Carraccio and colleagues noted that some sectors in medical education explored competency-based models in the 1970s. Elam laid down a series of principles and characteristics of CBET in 1971.

From these beginnings, interest within medical education began to grow. Competency-based models for medical education were soon promoted for wide use by McGaghie and colleagues as part of a report to **the World Health Organization (WHO)**[1] in 1978. In that report, the authors defined CBME as:

New Expressions

progression /prəˈɡreʃn/ n.（进入另一阶段的）发展；前进；进程

conception /kənˈsepʃn/ n. 构思；构想；设想

genesis /ˈdʒenəsɪs/ n. 开端；创始；起源

spur /spɜːr/ v. 促进，加速，刺激（某事发生）

---

① The text is adapted from the following source: Edgar, L. et al. 2000. *The Milestones Guidebook*. Chicago: American College of Graduate Medical Education.

 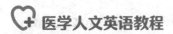

"The intended output of a competency-based program is a health professional who can practice medicine at a defined level of proficiency, in accord with local conditions, to meet local needs."

A group of international educators worked to "modernize" the definition of CBME and lay out the theoretical **rationale** for a CBME system. This group defined CBME as:

"an outcomes-based approach to the design, implementation, assessment and evaluation of a medical education program using an organizing framework of competencies."

Put simply, under CBME, graduation requirements and curricula would be based on standardized outcomes, while learning exercises and **formative** feedback would be personalized. While **momentum** was building for the principles and promises of CBME, there was also **consensus** that wide-spread acceptance would depend on addressing questions about:

- developing conceptual frameworks and language around CBME that would become well established and widely understood.

- designing learning outcomes, and with them, frameworks for assessment and evaluation.

- preparing faculty members to apply CBME principles in the learning environment.

- developing evidence that CBME produces better practitioners than the conventional approach.

A distinguishing feature of CBME is that learners could progress through the educational process at different rates: The most capable and talented individuals would be able to make career transitions earlier, while others would require more time (to a limit) to **attain** a sufficient level of knowledge, skills, and attitudes to enter unsupervised

New Expressions	
rationale /ˌræʃəˈnæl/ *n.* 基本原理；根本原因	**consensus** /kənˈsensəs/ *n.* 一致的意见；共识
formative /ˈfɔːrmətɪv/ *adj.* （对某事物或性格的发展）有重大影响的	**attain** /əˈteɪn/ *v.* （通常指经过努力）获得，得到
momentum /moʊˈmentəm/ *n.* 推进力；动力；势头	

practice. It is important to note that experience and time still matter in a CBME program, but time should not be treated as an intervention; rather, as a resource that should be used wisely and effectively. No one would argue that a certain quantity of experience is unimportant. Equally important are real system constraints in the United States that translate into the reality that the vast majority of graduate medical education (GME) programs would work in "**hybrid** models" of CBME—using competency-based educational principles in the context of fixed years of an educational program. A second key feature is the increased emphasis on assessment, especially ongoing, **longitudinal** assessment that enables faculty members to determine more accurately the developmental progress of the learner, as well as to help the learner through frequent feedback, coaching, and **adjustments** to learning plans. This is consistent with Anders Ericsson's work in **expertise** and deliberate practice, which demonstrates the need to tailor the educational experience to continually challenge the learner with experiences that are neither too easy nor overwhelming. Recent scholarship has **borne out** that frequent, actionable feedback about observable behaviors enables struggling residents to make improvements.

While defining the competencies was an important and necessary step, **operationalizing** and implementing them in practice prior to the **Milestones**[2] proved to be challenging. Program directors and faculty members struggled since the launch of the Outcome Project to understand what the competencies meant and, more importantly, what they should "look like" in practice. This lack of shared understanding **hampered** curricular changes, as well as development and evolution of better assessment methods. The challenges to operationalizing the competencies was not restricted to the United States, and during the last 18 years, several **notable** advancements have emerged in an effort to enable more effective implementation of CBME.

New Expressions	
hybrid /ˈhaɪbrɪd/ *n.*（不同事物的）混合物，合成物	**bear out** 证实；为……作证
longitudinal /ˌlɑːndʒəˈtuːdnl/ *adj.* 纵观的	**operationalize** /ˌɑpəˈreɪʃnəˌlaɪz/ *v.* 使开始运转；实施；使用于操作
adjustment /əˈdʒʌstmənt/ *n.*（行为、思想的）调整，适应	**hamper** /ˈhæmpər/ *v.* 妨碍；阻止；阻碍
expertise /ˌekspɜːrˈtiːz/ *n.* 专门知识；专门技能；专长	**notable** /ˈnoʊtəbl/ *adj.* 值得注意的；显著的；重要的

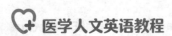
医学人文英语教程

Carraccio and colleagues described a four-step process for implementing CBME: (1) identification of the competencies; (2) determination of competency components and performance levels (e.g. benchmarks and milestones); (3) competency assessment; and (4) overall evaluation of the process. Similarly, Crawford and colleagues noted that individual programs would need to gain acceptance of their faculty members for CBME principles, offer faculty training in implementing CBME, and develop systems to assess trainee performance. Faculty members would need to develop skills in delivering timely and meaningful feedback to learners, and learners would need to assume "ownership" of their learning and familiarity with CMBE.

The consensus in current scholarship adds that the adoption of CBME practices increases when programs provide opportunities for stakeholder engagement and adaptation throughout the process. Adoption will take root in an organization when it is built upon a sound theory of what is to be accomplished, a clear connection between proposed practices and goals, and frequent opportunities for feedback, and course correction. Hall and his collaborators describe the initial identification of outcomes and design of assessment as a "sprint", while the long-term stakeholder engagement, learner buy-in, frequent evaluation, and modifications are the "marathon". In moving from implementation to adoption, Hall's program incorporated three-month and six-month reviews to ensure "fidelity" to the conceptual plans, and to enable faculty member and learner involvement.

Caverzagie and collaborators noted that buy-in and sharing of concepts would need to happen beyond individual programs. Wide-spread adoption would depend on aligning regulatory bodies around concepts of CBME; ensuring cooperation from programs, training locations, and health systems; and establishing methods of mutual accountability among the GME system and its stakeholders. Examples of such self-regulatory adoptions include the **ACGME**[3] Milestones and community

---

New Expressions

identification /aɪˌdentɪfɪˈkeɪʃn/ *n.* 确认；确定

adoption /əˈdɑːpʃn/ *n.* 采用（想法、计划、名字等）

stakeholder /ˈsteɪkhoʊldər/ *n.* （某组织、工程、体系等的）参与人，参与方；有权益关系者

adaptation /ˌædæpˈteɪʃn/ *n.* 适应

sprint /sprɪnt/ *n.* 短跑比赛；短距离速度竞赛

align /əˈlaɪn/ *v.* 使一致

accountability /əˌkaʊntəˈbɪləti/ *n.* （对自己的决定、行为）负有的责任，说明义务

created **entrustable** professional activities. These concepts approach competence as a developmental process and rely heavily on **positivist behavioral theory**[4].

New Expression

entrustable /ɪnˈtrʌstəbl/ *adj.* 可委托的

Notes

1. **the World Health Organization (WHO)**: 世界卫生组织。世界卫生组织是联合国机构，成立于 1948 年，以促进全球健康和控制疾病传播为主要目标，辅助会员国政府从事健康工作；在全世界有很多研究中心，进行生物医学研究；总部设在日内瓦。The World Health Organization is an agency of the United Nations. It was established in 1948 and aims to promote health and control communicable diseases. It assists in the efforts of member governments, and pursues biomedical research through all the collaborating research centers throughout the world. Its headquarters are in Geneva.

2. **Milestones**: 里程碑计划。里程碑计划是"胜任力导向的医学教育"模式的发展，旨在帮助医疗实践者成为更具有胜任力的医师，已经成为美国医学研究生教育的重要组成部分。里程碑计划围绕医师在六个胜任力领域应达到的技能、知识和行为水平进行了叙述性描述。The Milestones in GME provide narrative descriptors for the competencies and sub-competencies along a developmental continuum with varying degrees of granularity. Simply stated, the Milestones describe performance levels residents and fellows are expected to demonstrate for skills, knowledge, and behaviors in the six core competency domains.

3. **ACGME**: 研究生医学教育鉴定委员会。其全称是"Accreditation Council for Graduate Medical Education"。

4. **positivist behavioral theory**: 实证行为主义理论。positivist 指"实证主义的"。实证主义是由法国哲学家孔德在 19 世纪 30 年代开创的一个哲学流派。它从具体实在、可证实的东西出发，向人们提供实在、有用、确定、精确的知识。实证主义认为，感觉经验是真实知识的基础和出发点，超出经验的知识既不可靠，也不可知。behavioral theory 指"行为主义理论"，是由美国心理学家华生在巴甫洛夫条件反射学说的基础上创立的心理学理论，他主张心理学应该摒弃意识、意象等太多主观的东西，只研究所观察到的并能客观地加以测量的刺激和反应。Positivism is the

argument that we can learn things only through actually sensing them. This serves as the fundamental theoretical assumption of behaviorism, which only looks at the observable behaviors of subjects.

Post-reading Activities

I   Language Building-up

Task 1   Extensive Vocabulary Enlargement

Directions: *The following words are taken from the text. Please follow the three-step learning in this part and build up your own Extensive Vocabulary Chart.*

Step 1. Read through the words and underline them in the text. Circle the ones that are particularly new to you. Look up the words in the dictionary and put the equivalent Chinese translation in the chart below.

Step 2. While you go back to the text, please feel free to put any other words into the blanks provided in the extra lines in the chart.

Extensive Vocabulary Chart				
conception	formative	momentum	hybrid	longitudinal
adjustment	expertise	operationalize	hamper	notable
identification	stakeholder	adaptation	accountability	entrustable

Step 3. Please group the above words based on their parts of speech and meanings.

Nouns	

Verbs	
Adjectives	
Adverbs and Prepositions	
Medical Terminology	
Terminology in Other Fields	

Task 2　Intensive Vocabulary Enhancement

Directions: *The following 10 words are chosen from the text. They will form the intensive vocabulary in this unit. For intensive vocabulary, you are supposed to be able to explain them in English and use them in sentence and discourse constructions.*

Step 1. Please read through the words and be familiar with their Chinese and English definitions. Recall where and how they are used in the text.

Intensive Vocabulary Chart				
No.	Word	Translation	Definition	Status
1	progression	（进入另一阶段的）发展；前进；进程	*n.* the process of developing gradually from one stage or state to another	☆ ☆ ☆ ☆ ☆
2	rationale	基本原理；根本原因	*n.* the principles or reasons which explain a particular decision, course of action, belief, etc.	☆ ☆ ☆ ☆ ☆
3	genesis	开端；创始；起源	*n.* the beginning or origin of sth.	☆ ☆ ☆ ☆ ☆
4	spur	促进，加速，刺激（某事发生）	*v.* to make sth. happen faster or sooner	☆ ☆ ☆ ☆ ☆

Intensive Vocabulary Chart				
No.	Word	Translation	Definition	Status
5	consensus	一致的意见；共识	*n.* the opinion that all members of a group agree with	☆ ☆ ☆ ☆ ☆
6	attain	（通常指经过努力）获得，得到	*v.* to succeed in getting sth. usually after a lot of effort	☆ ☆ ☆ ☆ ☆
7	hamper	妨碍；阻止；阻碍	*v.* to prevent sb. from easily doing or achieving sth.	☆ ☆ ☆ ☆ ☆
8	adoption	采用（想法、计划、名字等）	*n.* the decision to start using sth., such as an idea, a plan, or a name	☆ ☆ ☆ ☆ ☆
9	sprint	短跑比赛；短距离速度竞赛	*n.* a race (e.g. a run, swim, etc.) in which people take part very fast over a short distance	☆ ☆ ☆ ☆ ☆
10	align	使一致	*v.* to change sth. slightly so that it is in the correct relationship to sth. else	☆ ☆ ☆ ☆ ☆

Step 2. Please tick the status for each word based on your own situation. If one word is very new or difficult for you, please tick five stars. Likewise, if one word is comparatively easy for you and you don't have to spend too much time on reading and learning it, then tick one star. The number of stars represents the difficulty of commanding a word in your eyes.

Step 3. Please complete the following 10 sentences by choosing appropriate words from the Intensive Vocabulary Chart. Please change the forms of the words where necessary.

1. The agreement is essential to _____ economic growth around the world.

   这项协议对于促进世界经济的增长至关重要。

2. His uncle is the world _____ champion.

   他的叔叔是短跑世界冠军。

3. Domestic prices have been _____ with those in world markets.

   国内价格已调整到与世界市场一致。

4. The _____ of new technology has improved the quality of life to a large extent.

   新技术的采用已经在很大程度上改善了生活质量。

5. We cannot yet satisfactorily explain the _____ of the universe.

   我们仍不能令人满意地解释宇宙的起源。

6. She is skilled at achieving _____ on sensitive issues.

   她擅长就敏感问题进行斡旋，从而达成共识。

7. What is the _____ behind these new exams?

   这些新考试的理论依据是什么？

8. Most of our students _____ five "A" grades in their exams.

   我们多数学生的考试成绩是五个优。

9. Kids at this stage will experience a natural _____ from childhood to adolescence.

   这个阶段的孩子会经历从童年到青少年的自然过渡。

10. Prejudice sometimes _____ a person from doing the right thing.

    有时候，偏见会妨碍人正确行事。

Task 3 Expressions and Sentences

Directions: *the following sentences are taken from the text. In each sentence, there is one phrase being underlined. Please refer to the dictionary and write down the explanation of the phrase in the line entitled "Meaning Exploration". After that, please make a sentence with it. Write the sentence in the line entitled "Sentence Making".*

Sentence 1

Original Sentence	Carraccio and colleagues noted that some sectors in medical education explored competency-based models in the 1970s. Elam laid down a series of principles and characteristics of CBET in 1971.
Meaning Exploration	lay down:
Sentence Making	

Sentence 2

Original Sentence	A group of international educators worked to "modernize" the definition of CBME and lay out the theoretical rationale for a CBME system.
Meaning Exploration	lay out:

Sentence Making	

Sentence 3

Original Sentence	Equally important are real system constraints in the United States that translate into the reality that the vast majority of graduate medical education (GME) programs would work in "hybrid models" of CBME...
Meaning Exploration	*translate into:*
Sentence Making	

Sentence 4

Original Sentence	Recent scholarship has borne out that frequent, actionable feedback about observable behaviors enables struggling residents to make improvements.
Meaning Exploration	*bear (sb./sth.) out:*
Sentence Making	

Sentence 5

Original Sentence	Adoption will take root in an organization when it is built upon a sound theory of what is to be accomplished, a clear connection between proposed practices and goals, and frequent opportunities for feedback, and course correction.
Meaning Exploration	*take root:*
Sentence Making	

Task 1 Overview and Comprehension

Directions: *The text could be divided into several different parts based on the subject matter it describes. Please summarize the main idea of the text by filling out the information in the chart below.*

Summary of the Main Content	
Origin of CBME	
Definition of CBME	
Components and Requirements of CBME	
Features of CBME	
The Process of Implementing CBME	

Task 2 Reflection and Discussion

Directions: *After reading, please reflect on the theme of the text. Work in groups and share your opinions on the following questions with other group members.*

According to the text, we know that both defining the "competencies" and operationalizing them in practice are key stages in CBME. As people from different contexts and cultures may have different understanding of "competencies" that a physician should acquire, these processes are bound to be challenging. What kind of competencies should be included in CBME? How should these competencies be measured and evaluated in different cultural contexts? Please reflect on these issues in relation to medical practices in China.

Part 3 Extended Reading

Medical Education Since World War I: Advances and Challenges①

After the **Flexner Report**, American medical education witnessed an institutional revolution. Medical schools exploded in size, wealth, and complexity. Resources were abundant, classes were smaller, and the average student received far more attention than students in the overflowing medical classes of Europe. Ever since American medical schools, universities, and teaching hospitals joined forces in the early 20th century, medical educators have seen their mission as a three-legged stool: education, research, and patient care. The stool, however, has not always been well balanced. Changes of professional power, economic climate, political support, and public trust have affected sources of funding and the relative priority of education.

The history of medical education since Flexner falls into three basic periods: In the first period, from the 1920s to the 1940s, medical schools saw themselves as primarily in the business of teaching; the needs of learners took precedence over research and patient care. Second, from World War II until the 1980s, research, fueled by the rapid growth of federal funds from the National Institutes of Health, replaced teaching as the most prestigious and valued aspect of medical schools. The final period, since the 1980s, witnessed the rise of managed care organizations and competition from corporate medicine and the need to generate income from faculty clinical practice, which reduced

New Expressions	
witness /'wɪtnəs/ v. 见证；是发生……的地点（或时间、组织等）	**climate** /'klaɪmət/ n. 倾向；思潮；风气；环境气氛
explode /ɪk'spləʊd/ v. 突增；激增	**federal** /'fedərəl/ adj.（在美国、加拿大等联邦制下）联邦政府的
abundant /ə'bʌndənt/ adj. 大量的；丰盛的；充裕的	**generate** /'dʒenəreɪt/ v. 产生；引起
stool /stuːl/ n. 凳子	

① The text is adapted from the following source: Cole, R. T. et al. 2015. *Medical Humanities: An Introduction*. New York: Cambridge University Press.

the funding and time available to educate students.

By the 1950s, medical schools had become an inseparable part of larger entities known as academic health centers. Although no two are alike, academic health centers are best understood as geographic complexes that contain a number of **contiguous**, collaborating institutions—medical schools, hospitals, research facilities, and other professional schools. They transformed medical education by linking it to the education of other health professionals and by **tying** education to large, **integrated** systems of health care delivery. By the 1990s, there were more than 125 academic health centers, but declining federal funding, **spiraling** health care costs, and a competitive health care market put many of them in financial **jeopardy**. The end of the 20th century has witnessed a second revolutionary period in American medical education, characterized by "the **erosion** of the clinical learning environment, the diminishing of faculty scholarship, and the reemergence of a **proprietary** system of medical schools in which the faculties' financial well-being was placed before education and research". The faculty who had previously been supported to teach and do research were told they had to devote their time to seeing increasing numbers of patients.

Despite these trends, reform-minded educators and scholars since the 1970s have **pressed** the case for respecting the patient as a whole person through active listening, **compassionate** presence, and **collaborative** decision-making. More recently, the need to educate and support the "whole student" has also become apparent. Evidence suggests that students, faculty, and physicians in general suffer from the financial pressures of academic health centers and the general **dehumanization** of modern medicine. These conditions contribute to significant rates of "**burnout**", a condition characterized by

New Expressions	
contiguous /kən'tɪɡjuəs/ *adj.* 相接的；相邻的	**press** /pres/ *v.* 坚持；反复强调
tie /taɪ/ *v.* 连接；联合；使紧密结合	**compassionate** /kəm'pæʃənət/ *adj.* 有同情心的；表示怜悯的
integrate /'ɪntɪɡreɪt/ *v.* 整合；（使）合并，成为一体	**collaborative** /kə'læbəreɪtɪv/ *adj.* 合作的；协作的；协力的
spiraling /'spaɪrəlɪŋ/ *adj.* 急剧上升的	**dehumanization** /ˌdiːˌhjuːmənə'zeɪʃn/ *n.* 去人性化
jeopardy /'dʒepərdi/ *n.* 危险；风险；危难	**burnout** /'bɜːrnaʊt/ *n.* 精疲力竭；倦怠
erosion /ɪ'roʊʒn/ *n.* 逐渐毁坏；削弱；损害	
proprietary /prə'praɪəteri/ *adj.* 专卖的；专营的；专利的	

emotional **exhaustion**, **depersonalization**, and decreased sense of self-efficacy. In response, programs for faculty health and well-being have sprung up, and self-care has become an important but still **underappreciated** concern for faculty and students alike.

In 2010, the Carnegie Foundation for the Advancement of Teaching—which sponsored the Flexner Report of 1910—published another major study of medical education in the United States. The new report named four key **deficiencies** in contemporary medical education. The first finding reveals the limits of the Flexnerian model a century after its adoption as medical training being "inflexible, overly long, and not learner-centered". A second finding described the poor **coordination** between excessive, formal "book" learning and experiential learning. The report's third finding noted the lack of **holistic** learning about patients' experiences and the absence of teaching about the "broader **civic** and **advocacy** roles of physicians". Finally, the report emphasized that the "pace and commercial nature of health care often impede the **inculcation** of fundamental values of the profession".

The new Carnegie Report is both a reflection of and an inspiration for a broad contemporary movement to reform medical education. It rightly calls for the **cultivation** of professional identity formation. It also advocates a better connection between formal knowledge and clinical experience; **facilitation** of lifelong learning and critical thinking; more flexible, individualized, and outcome-based ways to advance toward completion of a medical degree; and more engagement with population health, patient safety, and quality improvement.

Since the late 20th century, faculty and students—as well as patients—have become subject to damaging pressures in contemporary academic medicine and health care. Yet

---

New Expressions

exhaustion /ɪgˈzɔːstʃən/ n. 筋疲力尽；疲惫不堪

depersonalization /dɪˌpɜːrsənəlaɪˈzeɪʃn/ n. 人格解体；人性之丧失

underappreciated /ˌʌndərəˈpriːʃieɪtɪd/ adj. 不被赏识的

deficiency /dɪˈfɪʃnsi/ n. 缺点；缺陷

coordination /koʊˌɔːrdɪˈneɪʃn/ n. 协作；协调；配合

holistic /hoʊˈlɪstɪk/ adj. 整体的；全面的

civic /ˈsɪvɪk/ adj. 市政的；城市的；城镇的

advocacy /ˈædvəkəsi/ n.（对某思想、行动方针、信念的）拥护，支持，提倡

inculcation /ˌɪnkʌlˈkeɪʃn/ n. 反复灌输；谆谆教诲

cultivation /ˌkʌltɪˈveɪʃn/ n.（关系的）培植；（品质或技巧的）培养

facilitation /fəˌsɪlɪˈteɪʃn/ n. 促进

there are many encouraging responses, ranging from programs on faculty health and well-being to renewed emphasis on mentoring students and supporting development of their professional identity. Medical humanities attend to these issues by doing what it does best: facilitating active engagement with literature, history, ethics, art, and with spiritual resources. Topics, such as the ethics of health policy, the history of medicine, the experience of suffering, and the nature of healing help individuals address aspects of medicine and science where technical mastery is impossible, ethical problems are difficult, and **existential** meaning is hard to come by. Medical humanities allow students and faculty to reflect, **replenish,** and renew themselves. We suggest that humanizing patient care in the future will require recovering and supporting the humanity of students and faculty.

New Expressions

existential /ˌegzɪ'stenʃəl/ *adj.* 关于人类存在 的；与人类存在有关的   **replenish** /rɪ'plenɪʃ/ *v.* 补充；重新装满

Note

Flexner Report:《弗莱克斯纳报告》。该报告于 1910 年发布，引发了美国医学教育的剧烈变革，包括提高入学和学制标准，确立医学院教师的学术身份，配备实验室和教学医院，改变医学院运营的资金来源等。该报告极大地提高了西方医学教育的质量，促进了医学的职业化进程，使得医生成为精英职业，但也同时带来了低收入人群较难获得正规医疗服务等问题。The Flexner Report of 1910 transformed the nature and process of medical education in America with a resulting elimination of proprietary schools and the establishment of the biomedical model as the gold standard of medical training. This transformation occurred in the aftermath of the report, which embraced scientific knowledge and its advancement as the defining ethos of a modern physician.

Post-reading Activities

I Speaking Practice: Interview

Directions: *Please work in pairs. Imagine one of you is an interviewee, an experienced physician, and the other is an interviewer who is a first-year medical student at college. The purpose of the interview is to let the student get to know the profession better. Please design three interview questions and take turns to be the interviewer and the interviewee. You are welcome to design your questions based on the following piece of message taken from the text.*

> "... medical educators have seen their mission as a three-legged stool: education, research, and patient care. The stool, however, has not always been well balanced. Changes of professional power, economic climate, political support, and public trust have affected sources of funding and the relative priority of education."

Interview questions:

1. _____
2. _____
3. _____

II Reflective Writing Practice: Short Essay

Directions: *The text has outlined major developments of medical education since World War I. It is known that nowadays there are both opportunities and challenges facing medical education worldwide. Please think about the achievements and problems in Chinese medical education and write a reflective essay entitled "Medical Education in Contemporary China". The word limit is suggested to be 150–200 words.*

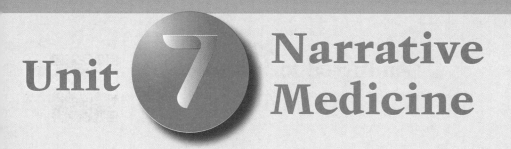

Unit 7 Narrative Medicine

> I used the phrase "narrative medicine" to refer to clinical practice fortified by narrative competence—the capacity to recognize, absorb, metabolize, interpret and be moved by the stories of illness.
>
> —Rita Charon

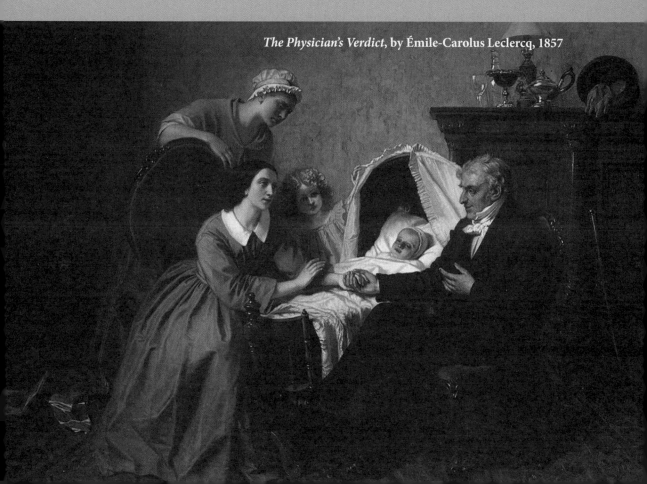

The Physician's Verdict, by Émile-Carolus Leclercq, 1857

Part 1 Academic Horizon

An Introduction to Narrative Medicine[①]

Narrative medicine began as a **rigorous** intellectual and clinical discipline to **fortify** health care with the capacity to skillfully receive the accounts persons give of themselves—to recognize, absorb, interpret, and be moved to action by the stories of others. It emerged to challenge the **reductionist**, **fragmented** medicine that holds little regard for the singular aspects of a patient's life and to protest the social injustice of a global health care system that **countenances** tremendous health disparities and **discriminatory** policies and practices. We clinicians, scholars, and creative writers who began this work together were convinced that narrative knowledge and skills have the power to improve health care by increasing the accuracy and scope of clinicians' knowledge of their patients and deepening the therapeutic partnerships they are able to form. The health care that recognizes and affiliates with patients, that exists to serve and not to profit, will **assure** justice while it promotes health for all.

From a **confluence** of narrative studies and clinical practices, we have developed an increasingly **nuanced** view of the workings of the narrative, relational, and reflexive

New Expressions	
rigorous /ˈrɪɡərəs/ *adj.* 谨慎的；细致的；彻底的	**countenance** /ˈkaʊntənəns/ *v.* 支持；赞成；同意
fortify /ˈfɔːrtɪfaɪ/ *v.* （在物质或精神上）加强，增强	**discriminatory** /dɪˈskrɪmɪnətɔːri/ *adj.* 区别对待的；不公正的；歧视的
reductionist /rɪˈdʌkʃənɪst/ *adj.* 简化论的；还原论的	**assure** /əˈʃʊr/ *v.* 使确信；向······保证
fragmented /fræɡˈmentɪd/ *adj.* 成碎片的；片断的；不完整的；四分五裂的	**confluence** /ˈkɑːnfluəns/ *n.* （事物的）汇合，汇聚，汇集
	nuanced /ˈnuːɑːnst/ *adj* 微妙的；具有细微差别的

---

① The text is adapted from the following source: Charon, R. et al. 2017. Introduction. In R. Charon et al. (Eds.), *The Principles and Practice of Narrative Medicine*. New York: Oxford University Press, 1–12.

processes of health care. **Literary theory**[1], **narratology**[2], **continental philosophies**[3], aesthetic theory, and cultural studies provide the intellectual foundations of narrative medicine. Informing our work are the 1980s' revolutionary upheavals in linguistic, narrative, and postmodern theory that led to profound questioning of certainty and a realization of language's ever-shifting representations of reality. Reading became recognized as an ethical act joining readers and writers in transformative engagement, leading to singular consequences for each reader instead of an orderly plotting toward an inevitable and shared conclusion. Primary care medicine, collaborative team-based health care, **narrative ethics**[4], the qualitative social science studies of health care, and psychoanalysis supply the clinical foundations of our work. From these sources come our commitments to relationships in patient-centered care and our conviction that narrative competence can widen the clinical gaze to include personal and social elements of patients' lives vital to the tasks of healing.

The goal of narrative medicine from its start has been to improve health care. We want to bring to clinical practice much that has been learned or hypothesized about the relationships between narrativity and identity, about the co-construction that takes place in any serious narrative telling, and about the discovery potential of creative acts. We want clinicians to come to appreciate the importance of the emotion and intersubjective relation borne of the telling and listening that occur in any clinical encounter. And we hope for patients that our work might open up health care to more trust, more accurate knowledge about one another, and more justice.

A group of scholars and clinicians teaching and practicing at **Columbia University**[5] in New York gathered at the millennium to take up questions that had engaged each of us in our work. Our inaugural efforts in narrative medicine began with questions of narrativity in the clinic: Why was it helpful for clinicians and trainees in health care

---

New Expressions

aesthetic /es'θetɪk/ *adj.* 审美的；有审美观点的；美学的

postmodern /ˌpoʊst'mɑːdərn/ *adj.* 后现代主义的

profound /prə'faʊnd/ *adj.* 艰深的；玄奥的

psychoanalysis /ˌsaɪkoʊə'næləsɪs/ *n.* 精神分析（或疗法）；心理分析（或疗法）

gaze /ɡeɪz/ *n.* 凝视；注视

hypothesize /haɪ'pɑːθəsaɪz/ *v.* 假设；假定

appreciate /ə'priːʃieɪt/ *v.* 理解；意识到；领会

intersubjective /ˌɪntərsəb'dʒektɪv/ *adj.* 主观间的；主体间的

clinical encounter 临床问诊

inaugural /ɪ'nɔːɡjərəl/ *adj.* 就职的；开幕的；成立的；创始的

to read and write? What **crystallized** was a dynamic and questing set of findings and concerns about the discovery nature of writing, the relational **substrate** of reading, the **affective** processes of narrating, the ethical complexities of the accounts of self, and how they all influence the wide ground of health. We early recognized attention, representation, and affiliation as the three movements of narrative medicine that emerged from our commitment to skilled listening, the power of representation to perceive the other, and the value of the partnerships that result from narrative contact. By attention we mean the state of heightened focus and commitment that a listener can donate to a teller—a patient, a student, a colleague, a friend. Rare, demanding, and rewarding, attention uses the listening self as a vessel to capture and reveal that which a teller has to tell. Representation, usually in writing but also in **visual** media, confers form on what is heard or perceived, thereby making it newly visible to both the listener and the teller. And affiliation, which results from deep attentive listening and the knowledge achieved through representation, binds patients and clinicians, students and teachers, self and other into relationships that support recognition and action as one stays the course with the other through whatever is to be faced.

One thing we have all consistently learned over the years is that clearings open up wherever we bring the methods of narrative medicine for teaching and learning. Not unlike the open spaces in a forest, these clearings function as sites of protection and safety, welcoming persons to join and work together without the **encumbrance** of hierarchy or status **differentials**. An **egality** that emits from storytelling itself levels even hard-bitten power **asymmetries**, so that members of interprofessional health care teams or groups of teachers and students or clinicians and patients can meet one another as equals, bent on reflexively giving and receiving, teaching and learning. Overtones, or **harmonics**, of care and unity are achievable in the health care that becomes a service at the command of patients rather than a professional **monopoly** that serves the interests

New Expressions	
crystallize /ˈkrɪstəlaɪz/ *v.* 变明确；使（想法、信仰等）明确	**differential** /ˌdɪfəˈrenʃl/ *n.* 差别；差额；差价；（尤指同行业不同工种的）工资级差
substrate /ˈsʌbstreɪt/ *n.* 底层；基底；基层	**egality** /iˈgæliti/ *n.* 均等；平等
affective /əˈfektɪv/ *adj.* 感情的；情感的	**asymmetry** /eˈsɪmɪtri/ *n.* 不对称；不对等
visual /ˈvɪʒuəl/ *adj.* 视力的；视觉的	**harmonic** /hɑːrˈmɑːnɪk/ *n.* 泛音
encumbrance /ɪnˈkʌmbrəns/ *n.* 妨碍者；累赘；障碍物	**monopoly** /məˈnɑːpəli/ *n.* 垄断；专营服务；被垄断的商品（或服务）

of the institutions who deliver it. All who seek care and all who seek to give care can unite in a clearing of safety, of purpose, of vision, and **unconditional** commitment to the interests of patients. This is the vision of narrative medicine.

New Expression

unconditional /ˌʌnkən'dɪʃənl/ *adj.* 无条件的；
无限制的；绝对的

Notes

1. **Literary theory**: 文学理论。文学理论是指诠释文学与文学批评的相关理论（或哲学）。各种文学理论派别会以不同的方式诠释、理解文学文本，并采用不同的研究方式来看待文学。Literary theory is the theory (or the philosophy) of the interpretation of literature and literary criticism.

2. **narratology**: 叙事学。叙事学是关于叙事、叙事结构及这两者如何影响我们知觉的理论及研究。Narratology refers to the branch of knowledge or criticism that deals with the structure and function of narrative and its themes, conventions, and symbols.

3. **continental philosophies**: 欧陆哲学。欧陆哲学指一些从欧洲大陆起源的相关哲学传统，与英美的分析哲学相对照。欧陆哲学包括现象学、存在主义、解释学、结构主义、后结构主义和后现代主义等。Continental philosophy is a set of 19th- and 20th-century philosophical traditions from the mainland of Europe. This sense of the term originated among English-speaking philosophers in the second half of the 20th century, who used it to refer to a range of thinkers and traditions outside the analytic movement.

4. **narrative ethics**: 叙事伦理。叙事伦理的核心概念主要包括：（1）每一个伦理情境都是独一无二、不可重复的，普适性原则无法获得每个伦理情境的全部意义；（2）在任何一个与健康相关的情境中，评判任何决定或行动是否恰当的标准是看它是否与病人的个人生命故事相一致。The central tenets of narrative ethics are as follows: (1) Every moral situation is unique and unrepeatable and its meaning cannot be fully captured by appealing to law like universal principles; (2) In any given health care situation, any decision or course of action is justified in terms of its fit with the individual life story or stories of the patient.

5. **Columbia University**: 哥伦比亚大学。Columbia University is a university in New York City, one of the most prestigious universities in the United States. It was founded in 1754.

Post-reading Activities

I Speaking Practice: Group Discussion

Directions: *Please discuss the following questions in small groups. After your discussion, please share your opinions with the whole class.*

1. What ideas would come to your mind when you hear the term "narrative medicine"? What is your understanding of the origin and definition of narrative medicine?

2. What is the goal of narrative medicine and what are the means to realize the goal?

3. What is known about the three movements of narrative medicine?

4. Have you been to the hospital as a patient? What are your best and worst experiences of communicating with doctors?

II Speaking Practice: Oral Presentation

Directions: *The following remark is taken from the text. Please talk about your understanding and opinion of it. Do you agree with the author's opinion? Under what circumstances will the "harmonics of care and unity" become achievable? What are the differences between the two kinds of health care services mentioned in the remark? Please feel free to use examples either from your daily life experiences or from medical movies or dramas to illustrate your ideas.*

"Overtones, or harmonics, of care and unity are achievable in the health care that becomes a service at the command of patients rather than a professional monopoly that serves the interests of the institutions who deliver it."

Part 2 Thematic Reading

Why Narrative Medicine Is Committed to Close Reading[①]

In an essay in the 2007 Modern Language Association's *Profession*, **feminist** scholar **Jane Gallop**[1] writes that "**Close reading**[2]... learned through practice with literary texts, learned in literature classes, is a widely applicable skill, of value not just to scholars in other disciplines but to a wide range of students with many different futures. Students trained in close reading have been known to apply it to diverse sorts of texts—newspaper articles, textbooks in other disciplines, political speeches—and thus to discover things they would not otherwise have noticed."

If close reading helps persons "to discover things they would not otherwise have noticed", perhaps it might help clinicians to notice what their patients try to tell them. The close reader, as **Jane Tompkins**[3] suggests, becomes gradually more receptive to appreciating texts outside of the literature class. She continues: "This enhanced, intensified reading can prove **invaluable** for many kinds of jobs as well as in their lives." **Transcending** the conventional boundaries of close reading, narrative medicine reading practices reach beyond literary texts to examine and try to understand visual and musical arts, personal conversations, the mood in a room, or the silent communication of performance and gesture.

New Expressions	
feminist /'femənɪst/ *adj.*（有关）女权主义的；支持女权运动的	**transcend** /træn'send/ *v.* 超出，超越（通常的界限）
invaluable /ɪn'væljuəbl/ *adj.* 极有用的；极宝贵的	

---

① The text is adapted from the following source: Charon, R. et al. 2017. Close reading: The signature method of narrative medicine. In R. Charon et al. (Eds.), *The Principles and Practice of Narrative Medicine*. New York: Oxford University Press, 157–179.

The **dividends** for narrative medicine in close reading are found in those features that distinguish it from casual, technical, or information-seeking reading. The close reader absorbs a text, **squandering** nothing. Whether reading a novel, a lyric poem, or a paper in *JAMA*[4], he or she notes the **genre**, the **diction**, the **temporal** structure, the spaces depicted, and the **metaphorical** and musical work being done with the words. The close reader registers who is telling the text's story—whether a first-person or third-person narrator, whether or not this narrator is involved in the action of the plot, whether remote, familiar, reliable, inviting, or **combative**. The close reader appreciates the text's **meter** and rhythm; he or she recognizes when the text **alludes** to some other text outside of itself. As if in conversation with the author, the reader is aware of his or her own place in the text, asking questions about the contract with the author that emerges from the text. What duty, the reader asks in the key of narrative ethics, do "I" **incur** by reading this book?

Close reading thickens and complicates the effects of the words on the page. The text is treated as a thing of beauty, an occasion of **bliss**, a created object of both rare delicacy and raw power. **Alternatively**, it might be experienced as **noxious**, **revolting**, **denigrating** of values held closely by the reader. Or it may be received with indifference, the reader **impervious**, despite effort, to the forces of the text. Sometimes a reader encounters a book he or she does not want to be inhabited by. Literary critic **Wayne Booth**[5], who championed the field of ethical criticism, **emphatically** reserves the right of any reader to refuse to become the kind of reader being demanded by a particular book. You simply close the book. All of these aspects of the text contribute to its **ultimate**

New Expressions	
dividend /ˈdɪvɪdend/ *n.* 红利，股息，股利（引申为：好处；厚报）	**incur** /ɪnˈkɜːr/ *v.* 引致，带来（成本、花费等）
squander /ˈskwɑːndər/ *v.* 浪费，挥霍（金钱、时间等）	**bliss** /blɪs/ *n.* 完美的愉悦感；欣喜
genre /ˈʒɑːnrə/ *n.* （文学、艺术、电影或音乐的）体裁，类型	**alternatively** /ɔːlˈtɜːrnətɪvli/ *adv.* （引出第二种选择或可能的建议）要不，或者
diction /ˈdɪkʃn/ *n.* 措辞；用语；用词	**noxious** /ˈnɑːkʃəs/ *adj.* 有毒的；有害的
temporal /ˈtempərəl/ *adj.* 时间的	**revolting** /rɪˈvoʊltɪŋ/ *adj.* 令人作呕的；极其讨厌的
metaphorical /ˌmetəˈfɔːrɪkl/ *adj.* 隐喻的；含比喻的；比喻性的	**denigrate** /ˈdenɪɡreɪt/ *v.* 诋毁；诽谤；贬低
combative /kəmˈbætɪv/ *adj.* 好斗的；好争论的	**impervious** /ɪmˈpɜːrviəs/ *adj.* 不受影响的
meter /ˈmiːtər/ *n.* （诗歌的）韵律，格律	**emphatically** /ɪmˈfætɪkəli/ *adv.* 强调地；断然地；明显地
allude /əˈluːd/ *v.* 间接提到；暗指；影射	**ultimate** /ˈʌltɪmət/ *adj.* 最后的；最终的；终极的

meaning—for this one reader—and help to expose what this reader undergoes by virtue of reading it.

We have shown at Columbia University that rigorous close reading can be taught and learned in clinical settings, where its dividends have been found to enhance patient care. But teaching health care professionals how to be close readers does far more than improve their interviewing skills. Here is where we find the transformative potential of our practice of narrative medicine. The close reader gradually discovers that the world within the text—be it a novel, a newspaper story, one's own diary, or an account of illness given by a patient in the **emergency room**—is real. The creative acts of representation—in writing or telling or painting or composing—do not merely reflect something real but create something real. A work of art results in a product, not a copy. Radical, disturbing, a challenge to reductive objectivity, the realization of the createdness of the real by and in language can shock the unprepared newcomer to the acts of reading. Rigorous training in close reading—at least narrative medicine's version of close reading—improves readers' capacity for attention but also **revolutionizes** the reader's position in life from being an **onlooker** checking the log of past events to becoming a daring participant in the emergence of reality. The trainee comes to realize that, until told or written or in some way represented, events remain unheard, **unconfigured**, and therefore **imperceptible**. Such **unformed chaotic** experiences will not allow themselves to be known. But once configured by language or an image or composition, once form has been conferred onto the unformed, the chaos is discernible both by those who witness it and those who hear accounts of it. Once represented, the chaos is at least potentially comprehensible. It will then have been recognized.

Close reading became one of the narrative medicine's foundational methods for its teaching and practice because it serves all the various uses of the reader's skill. For sure, close reading prepares a student to read complex literary texts with attention and skill and even to read or hear accounts of illness with nuance and sophisticated

New Expressions	
emergency room （医院）急诊室	**imperceptible** /ˌɪmpər'septəbl/ adj. （小得）无法察觉的，感觉不到的
revolutionize /ˌrevə'luːʃənaɪz/ v. 彻底改变；完全变革	
onlooker /'ɔːnlʊkər/ n. 旁观者	**unformed** /ˌʌn'fɔːrmd/ adj. 发展不充分的；未成形的；不成熟的
unconfigured /ˌʌnkən'fɪɡjərd/ adj. 未配置的	**chaotic** /keɪ'ɑːtɪk/ adj. 混乱的；杂乱的；紊乱的

comprehension. At the same time, it fulfills a far more **weighty** duty. It not only suggests but demonstrates that one's acts as a person who cares for the sick arise from the same "self" as that person who is transported by a **Rothko**[6] painting, a **Bach partita**[7], or a novel by **Virginia Woolf**[8]. The close reader becomes, in the end, more deeply and powerfully **attuned** to all that may lie in awareness and outside of awareness, in consciousness and out of consciousness, in body, in mind, and whatever is left once those two are accounted for; in relation to the voice and the presence of the other. Close reading may be a **threshold** to a life fully lived.

New Expressions

weighty /'weɪti/ *adj.* 严重的；重要的；重大的　　**threshold** /'θreʃhəʊld/ *n.* 开端；起点；入门
attune /ə'tjuːn/ *v.* 使协调；使合拍；使适应

Notes

1. **Jane Gallop:** 简·盖洛普，1952年至今；美国威斯康星大学密尔沃基分校英语与比较文学教授。Jane Gallop is an American professor who since 1992 has served as Distinguished Professor of English and Comparative Literature at the University of Wisconsin-Milwaukee, where she has taught since 1990.

2. **Close reading:** 文本细读法。In literary criticism, the term "close reading" describes the careful, sustained interpretation of a brief passage of a text. Close reading emphasizes the single and the particular over the general, effected by close attention to individual words, the syntax, and the order in which the sentences unfold ideas, as a reader scans the line of the text.

3. **Jane Tompkins:** 简·汤普金斯，1940年至今。Jane Tompkins is a professor of English at Duke University. She is the author of *Reader-Response Criticism*, which remains an indispensable guide to reader-response criticism.

4. *JAMA*:《美国医学会杂志》。*The Journal of the American Medical Association (JAMA)*, published continuously since 1883, is an international peer-reviewed general medical journal.

5. **Wayne Booth:** 韦恩·布斯，1921—2005；美国著名文学评论家。Wayne Booth was an American literary critic. He was the George M. Pullman Distinguished Service Professor Emeritus in English Language and Literature at the University of

Chicago. His work followed largely from the Chicago school of literary criticism.

6. **Rothko:** 罗思科，1903—1970；美国画家，大色域绘画的主要人物。Rothko was a U.S. painter and a leading figure in color-field painting.

7. **Bach partita:** 巴赫变奏曲。约翰·塞巴斯蒂安·巴赫（Johann Sebastian Bach），1685—1750，巴洛克时代晚期的德国作曲家和管风琴家，历史上最伟大的作曲家之一。Johann Sebastian Bach was a German composer and organist of the late baroque period, who was also one of the greatest composers in history. Partita was originally the name for a single-instrumental piece of music (in the 16th and 17th centuries), but Johann Kuhnau (Thomaskantor until 1722) and his successor Johann Sebastian Bach used it for collections of musical pieces, as a synonym for the dance suite.

8. **Virginia Woolf:** 弗吉尼亚·伍尔芙，1882—1941；英国小说家和评论家。Virginia Woolf was an English writer and one of the foremost modernists of the 20th century.

Post-reading Activities

I **Language Building-up**

Task 1 Extensive Vocabulary Enlargement

Directions: *The following words are taken from the text. Please follow the three-step learning in this part and build up your own Extensive Vocabulary Chart.*

Step 1. Read through the words and underline them in the text. Circle the ones that are particularly new to you. Look up the words in the dictionary and put the equivalent Chinese translation in the chart below.

Step 2. While you go back to the text, please feel free to put any other words into the blanks provided in the extra lines in the chart.

Extensive Vocabulary Chart				
dividend	squander	diction	metaphorical	meter

Extensive Vocabulary Chart				
allude	incur	bliss	alternatively	noxious
revolting	denigrate	impervious	emphatically	ultimate
unconfigured	unformed	chaotic	weighty	attune

Step 3. Please group the above words based on their parts of speech and meanings.

Nouns	
Verbs	
Adjectives	
Adverbs and Prepositions	
Medical Terminology	
Terminology in Other Fields	

Directions: *The following 10 words are chosen from the text. They will form the intensive vocabulary in this unit. For intensive vocabulary, you are supposed to be able to explain them in English and use them in sentence and discourse constructions.*

Step 1. Please read through the words and be familiar with their Chinese and English definitions. Recall where and how they are used in the text.

No.	Word	Translation	Definition	Status
		Intensive Vocabulary Chart		
1	feminist	（有关）女权主义的；支持女权运动的	*adj.* of, relating to, or supporting feminism	☆ ☆ ☆ ☆ ☆
2	invaluable	极有用的；极宝贵的	*adj.* extremely useful	☆ ☆ ☆ ☆ ☆
3	transcend	超出，超越（通常的界限）	*v.* to be or go beyond the usual limits of sth.	☆ ☆ ☆ ☆ ☆
4	genre	（文学、艺术、电影或音乐的）体裁；类型	*n.* a particular type or style of literature, art, film, or music that sb. can recognize because of its special features	☆ ☆ ☆ ☆ ☆
5	temporal	时间的	*adj.* connected with or limited by time	☆ ☆ ☆ ☆ ☆
6	combative	好斗的；好争论的	*adj.* ready and willing to fight or argue	☆ ☆ ☆ ☆ ☆
7	revolutionize	彻底改变；完全变革	*v.* to completely change the way that sth. is done	☆ ☆ ☆ ☆ ☆
8	onlooker	旁观者	*n.* a person who watches sth. that is happening but is not involved in it	☆ ☆ ☆ ☆ ☆
9	imperceptible	（小得）无法察觉的，感觉不到的	*adj.* very small and therefore unable to be seen or felt	☆ ☆ ☆ ☆ ☆
10	threshold	开端；起点；入门	*n.* the point just before a new situation, period of life, etc. begins	☆ ☆ ☆ ☆ ☆

Step 2. Please tick the status for each word based on your own situation. If one word is very new or difficult for you, please tick five stars. Likewise, if one word is comparatively easy for you and you don't have to spend too much time on reading and learning it, then tick one star. The number of stars represents the difficulty of commanding a word in your eyes.

Step 3. Please complete the following 10 sentences by choosing appropriate words from the Intensive Vocabulary Chart above. Please change the forms of the words where necessary.

1. Their advice was _____ to me at that stage of my work.

2. He made some enemies with his _____ style.

3. His work _____ the treatment of this disease.

4. The present world crisis should in principle be analyzed from different _____ _____ perspectives.

5. Jenny is a fervent supporter of the _____ movement.

6. She was on the _____ of a dazzling career.

7. The desire for peace _____ political differences.

8. Such changes are _____ to even the best-trained eye.

9. The novel and short story are different _____.

10. A crowd of _____ had gathered at the scene of the accident.

Task 3 Expressions and Sentences

Directions: *The following sentences are taken from the text. In each sentence, there is one phrase being underlined. Please refer to the dictionary and write down the explanation of the phrase in the line entitled "Meaning Exploration". After that, please make a sentence with it. Write the sentence in the line entitled "Sentence Making".*

Sentence 1

Original Sentence	Students trained in close reading have been known to apply it to diverse sorts of texts…
Meaning Exploration	*apply... to...:*
Sentence Making	

Sentence 2

Original Sentence	The dividends for narrative medicine in close reading are found in those features that distinguish it from casual, technical, or information-seeking reading.
Meaning Exploration	*distinguish... from...:*

Sentence Making	

Sentence 3

Original Sentence	As if in conversation with the author, the reader is aware of his or her own place in the text, asking questions about the contract with the author that emerges from the text.
Meaning Exploration	*be aware of:*
Sentence Making	

Sentence 4

Original Sentence	All of these aspects of the text contribute to its ultimate meaning—for this one reader—and help to expose what this reader undergoes by virtue of reading it.
Meaning Exploration	*by virtue of:*
Sentence Making	

Sentence 5

Original Sentence	Once represented, the chaos is at least potentially comprehensible.
Meaning Exploration	*at least:*
Sentence Making	

II Critical Reading and Thinking

Task 1 Overview and Comprehension

Directions: *While reading an article, it is a good habit to take down some reading notes. Reading notes usually include the main idea and key information provided in* *the article. Please read through the text and provide the missing information in the following Reading Notes.*

Reading Notes	
Benefits of Close Reading	
Features of Close Reading	
Close Reading as One of the Narrative Medicine's Foundational Methods	

Task 2　Reflection and Discussion

Directions: *After reading, please reflect on the theme of the text. Work in groups and share your opinions on the following questions with other group members.*

1. What might we gain from close reading according to Jane Gallop?
2. What are the features of close reading which distinguish it from casual, technical, or information-seeking reading?
3. Why did close reading become one of the narrative medicine's foundational methods for its teaching and practice?
4. From your point of view, how can you translate the skills acquired in the close reading of literary works to clinical practice with the aim of improving health care communication with patients?

医学人文英语教程

Part 3 Extended Reading

A Place of Memory and Learning[①]

René Leriche[1] famously wrote, "Every surgeon carries within himself a small **cemetery**, where from time to time he goes to pray—a place of bitterness and regret, where he must look for an explanation for his failures." Instead of a cemetery in my head, I have a 1.5-inch binder that lives above my desk. Within the binder is a single page for every one of my patients who has died. The collection is not a place of bitterness and regret. Instead, it is a place I visit to pay my respects, to learn, to **reminisce**, and to observe the **arc** of my career.

I started this collection in 1997 when the first patient I cared for as an **attending** primary care physician died. After I hung up the phone with the patient's brother, I looked at the "face sheet" and wondered what to do with it. The single hand-written page included the patient's name, date of birth, medical record number, problem list, and other notes about the case. I could not bear to **discard** it so I placed it in a drawer. Over the years, I laid additional sheets on top of it. Years later, when I emptied my office for a move, I was surprised by the thickness of the **stack** of pages. I placed them, maintaining their **chronological** order, into a half inch binder.

That first patient came to me for an initial visit having lost 50 pounds. On examination, I discovered the largest, hardest, **supraclavicular** node I had ever felt.

New Expressions	
cemetery /'semətəri/ n.（尤指不靠近教堂的）墓地，坟地，公墓	**stack** /stæk/ n.（通常指码放整齐的）一叠，一摞，一堆
reminisce /ˌremɪ'nɪs/ v. 回忆，追忆，缅怀（昔日的快乐时光）	**chronological** /ˌkrɑːnə'lɑːdʒɪkl/ adj. 按发生时间顺序排列的
arc /ɑːrk/ n. 弧形	**supraclavicular** /ˌsuprəklə'vɪkjələr/ adj. 锁骨上的
attending /ə'tendɪŋ/ adj.（医生）主治的	
discard /dɪs'kɑːrd/ v. 丢弃；抛弃	

① The text is adapted from the following source: Cifu, A. S. 2021. A place of memory and learning. *JAMA, 325*(19): 1939–1940.

When the **cytopathologist** arrived to perform a needle aspiration of the mass, he was unable to penetrate it with the needle. Fresh out of training, at a time when "unnecessary **hospitalization**" was **anathematic**, I managed the patient's care as an **outpatient**. Twenty-five years later, I would have managed the case differently.

Over the years, what I have added to the binder has changed. The face sheets have gone from hand-written ones to **printouts** from one and then another electronic medical record system. I have added the cause of death, circling the entry on the problem list that had progressed to a fatal illness or adding a new diagnosis when the end was sudden and unexpected. I occasionally **staple** other **mementos**, such as **obituaries**, to the entries. Sometimes I **jot** down reflections. Every ten or so years I buy a thicker binder—first 1 inch, most recently 1.5 inches.

When I realized that this collection was something that I was going to maintain, I added one more sheet to the very back. This page was for the first patient of mine who died. I cared for him in my resident continuity clinic, and he died during my **residency**. He was a young man, whom I still remember for his quiet, gentlemanly manner. He died of AIDS-related complications, an all-too-common cause in the pre-**HAART**[2] era. Had he lived another couple of years, we could have offered effective therapy for his HIV.

Although I do not see my collection as **morbid**, I do worry that my colleagues and trainees who learn of it might. Activities like this one are not foreign to me. I am a collector. I am also a **sentimentalist** who **whiles away** hours looking through boxes of pictures and family **memorabilia**. The binder entries **memorialize** people with whom I was, however briefly, closely associated. I spent time with them and with their families. I

New Expressions	
cytopathologist /ˌsaɪtəʊpə'θɑːlədʒɪst/ *n.* 细胞病理学家	**jot** /dʒɑːt/ *v.* 草草记下；匆匆记下
hospitalization /ˌhɑːspɪtələ'zeɪʃn/ *n.* 住院治疗	**residency** /'rezɪdənsi/ *n.* 高级专科住院医生实习期
anathematic /əˌnæθə'mætɪk/ *adj.* 厌恶的	**morbid** /'mɔːrbɪd/ *adj.* 病态的；不正常的
outpatient /'aʊtpeɪʃnt/ *n.* 门诊病人	**sentimentalist** /ˌsentɪ'mentəlɪst/ *n.* 好感伤者；多愁善感的人
printout /'prɪntaʊt/ *n.* （计算机）打印件；打印资料	**while away** 逍遥自在地度过；消磨（时间）
staple /'steɪpl/ *v.* 用订书钉装订	**memorabilia** /ˌmemərə'bɪliə/ *n.* 收藏品；纪念品
memento /mə'mentoʊ/ *n.* 纪念品	**memorialize** /mə'mɔːriəlaɪz/ *v.* 纪念
obituary /oʊ'bɪtʃueri/ *n.* 讣闻；讣告	

often woke up in the middle of the night thinking about them. Unlike my own deceased relatives, however, these are people I have no other way of remembering. I cannot share stories about them over a family dinner.

Thumbing through the pages I am struck by how medicine and my clinical practice have changed. In the early years, there are deaths from AIDS, heart disease, and **emphysema**. As I thumb from the earliest entries to the middle years, cancer deaths become most common. This evolution probably reflects improved care of HIV and **cardiovascular** disease and declining rates of smoking as well as the general "aging" of my patient panel. When I look over the most recent years, at least half the patients died after falls or causes that I can only identify as "old age"—when everything went wrong.

The **ephemera** that I sometimes attach to the face sheets have also changed over the years. The early pages have nothing attached. These were patients I knew only briefly. As those who died had been with me for longer periods, their entries are often **adorned** with death notices, prayer cards, and funeral invitations. As the people who joined my practice changed, additions of long obituaries from local and national papers appear. Most treasured are the thank-you notes, usually written by a **grieving** family member. Two pages have attached notes written by the patients themselves, penned during their final days. These left me speechless.

While the first two entries in the binder are permanent, the final one is always **temporary**; its place soon taken by a more recently deceased patient. Right now, this position is taken by a patient who died far too young. This person was a peer of mine— a professional who shared with me a similar education and upbringing. Though our relationship lasted only a few years, we grew remarkably close. Despite the team of physicians involved, it was always me this person consulted with before making treatment decisions. It was also me that the patient came to when it was time to initiate hospices.

New Expressions	
deceased /dɪ'siːst/ *adj.* 死去了的；已死的；亡故的	**ephemera** /ɪ'femərə/ *n.* 只在短期内有用的事物
thumb through 快速翻阅	**adorn** /ə'dɔːrn/ *v.* 装饰；装扮
emphysema /ˌemfɪ'siːmə/ *n.* 肺气肿	**grieve** /griːv/ *v.* （尤指因某人的去世而）悲伤，悲痛，伤心
cardiovascular /ˌkɑːrdioʊ'væskjələr/ *adj.* 心血管的	**temporary** /'tempəreri/ *adj.* 短暂的；暂时的；临时的

There is pain in this binder. Every name is familiar, but there are many about whom I recall nothing else. That evidence of our impermanence saddens me. There are names that recall anxiety, family meetings that could have gone better, tears and anger in examination rooms, and guilt about times I believe I fell short.

What will I do with this binder when I stop practicing medicine? Given my history with it, I expect it will be one of the few physical objects I take with me. I will leave with the memories and lessons of the patients who died on my watch. My living patients will go on to form new relationships with others who will be responsible for caring for them while they live, and remembering them when they are gone.

New Expression
impermanence /ɪmˈpɜːrmənəns/ *n.* 暂时性； 无常

Notes

1. **René Leriche:** 雷内·勒里奇，1879—1955；法国著名外科医生。勒里奇于 1917 年实施了第一例动脉周围交感神经切除术并获得成功，在现代外科史上有着重要的地位。Leriche was a renowned French surgeon who held a significant position in modern surgical history. In 1917, he successfully performed the first sympathectomy, the surgery involving the removal of the sympathetic nerves surrounding arteries.

2. **HAART:** 高效抗逆转录病毒治疗。The use of multiple drugs that act on different viral targets is known as highly active antiretroviral therapy (HAART). HAART decreases the patients' total burden of HIV, maintains function of the immune system, and prevents opportunistic infections that often lead to death.

Post-reading Activities

I Speaking Practice: Interview

Directions: *Please work in pairs. Imagine one of you is an interviewee, the author of the article "A Place of Memory and Learning", and the other is an interviewer who interviews the author about his experience of being a doctor. Please design three interview questions and take turns to be the interviewer and the interviewee.*

Interview questions:

1. _____

2. _____

3. _____

II Reflective Writing Practice: Short Essay

Directions: *René Leriche said "Every surgeon carries within himself a small cemetery, where from time to time he goes to pray—a place of bitterness and regret, where he must look for an explanation for his failures." Please think about doctors' experiences of success and failure in their daily medical practices and write a reflective essay entitled "What Can Doctors Learn from Their Patients?". Please use concrete examples to illustrate your ideas. The word limit is suggested to be 150–200 words.*

Unit 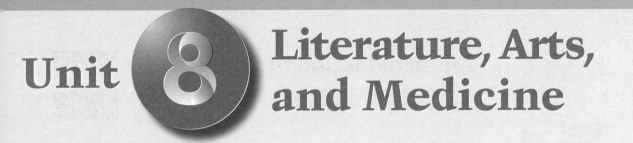 8 Literature, Arts, and Medicine

> *All sorrows can be borne if you put them into a story or tell a story about them.*
>
> *—Isak Dinesen*

Unconscious Patient (Allegory of Smell),
by Rembrandt Harmenszoon van Rijn, 1924–1925

Part 1 Academic Horizon

An Introduction to Literature, Arts, and Medicine[1]

The term "the arts" **derives** its meaning from the context in which it is used. "**Fine arts**[1]" refers to activities and products of the imagination, such as music, painting, and sculpture, which appeal to a sense of beauty. Branches of learning, such as history, languages, literature, philosophy, and religion are traditionally known in academic **parlance** as **liberal arts**[2]. "Arts and sciences" distinguishes the humanities, also known as human sciences, from natural sciences and social sciences. Similarly, in an older idiom, "letters and sciences" draws the same distinction but gives literary learning pride of place in the humanities. And there are "arts of", as in **martial arts** and healing arts. In this article, we will try to explore some contemporary connections between humanistic study and the healing arts, and the relationships between visual and **verbal** meaning.

Art both **mirrors** and challenges our settled perceptions. **John Berger**[3] (1972) writes, "Seeing comes before words... (and) the way we see things is affected by what we know or what we believe. We only see what we look at. To look is an act of choice. As a result of this act, what we see is brought within our reach."

Conversely, visual images also shape the way we think. Being **bombarded** with images, as we are, is not **conducive** to reflection. Pausing to look questioningly at a

New Expressions	
derive /dɪˈraɪv/ v. (从……中) 得到，获得	**mirror** /ˈmɪrər/ v. 反映
parlance /ˈpɑːrləns/ n. 用语；术语	**bombard** /bɑːmˈbɑːrd/ v. 轰击；轰炸
martial /ˈmɑːrʃl/ adj. 战争的；军事的	**conducive** /kənˈduːsɪv/ adj. 使容易（或有可能）发生的
martial arts 武术	
verbal /ˈvɜːrbl/ adj. 文字的；言语的；词语的	

① The text is adapted from the following sources: Cole, R. T. et al. 2015. *Medical Humanities: An Introduction*. New York: Cambridge University Press.

Charon, R. et al. 1995. Literature and medicine: Contributions to clinical practice. *Annals of Internal Medicine, 122*(8): 600.

 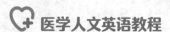

painting or photograph, or to critically view a film or television show prompts us to think more deeply about what we are seeing.

In a discussion of her experience teaching medical students utilizing a range of visual materials, Mary Winkler (1993) describes how asking students to look carefully at "artworks that treat such subjects as death, pain, aging, fear, bureaucratic indifference, and poverty", and then asking them to consider the question "What do you see?" elicits empathy and "reinforces the idea of our common humanity and the vulnerability that we all share". You will find images in literature, painting, and films that encourage you to reflect, probe for deeper meanings, and articulate personal reactions.

As with images, the written word, too, can shape us by inclining us to introspection and circumspection and by inviting us into the lives of others. Reading narratives of illness and stories of doctoring extends the reach of our minds and sensibilities, and deepens fellow feeling. This is important because, as **Clifford Geertz**[4] observes, "the reach of our minds, the range of signs we can manage somehow to interpret, is what defines the intellectual, emotional, and moral space in which we live". Vicariously experiencing, through the prism of poetry and the medium of memoirs, what others have been through illuminates that space and makes it more capacious. We know more and understand more fully for having experienced, at one remove, what it is like to hurt or heal.

What is more, we gain self-knowledge at the level of feeling. According to **Cameron**[5], "The power and charm of the arts is that in them we discover the life of feeling that might sleep in us unregarded without their help... It is as though we don't understand our own feelings until we are confronted with a contrived state of affairs

New Expressions	
bureaucratic /ˌbjʊrə'krætɪk/ *adj.* 官僚的；官僚主义的	**vicariously** /vaɪ'keɪriəsli/ *adv.* 间接感受到地
elicit /ɪ'lɪsɪt/ *v.* 引出	**prism** /'prɪzəm/ *n.* 棱镜；三棱镜
empathy /'empəθi/ *n.* 同感；共鸣；同情；共情	**medium** /'miːdiəm/ *n.*（传播信息的）媒介，手段，方法
articulate /ɑːr'tɪkjuleɪt/ *v.* 明确表达；清楚说明	**illuminate** /ɪ'luːmɪneɪt/ *v.* 照明；照亮；照射
incline /ɪn'klaɪn/ *v.*（使）倾向于；有……的趋势	**capacious** /kə'peɪʃəs/ *adj.* 容量大的；容积大的；宽敞的
introspection /ˌɪntrə'spekʃn/ *n.* 反省；内省	
circumspection /ˌsɜːrkəm'spekʃn/ *n.* 小心谨慎；考虑周密；慎重	**at one remove** 通过别人的体验来感受
	unregarded /ˌʌnrɪ'gɑːrdɪd/ *adj.* 不受注意的
sensibility /ˌsensə'bɪləti/ *n.*（尤指文艺方面的）感受能力，鉴赏力；敏感性	**contrived** /kən'traɪvd/ *adj.* 预谋的；不自然的；人为的

that isn't a direct **rendering** of our feelings but somehow expresses their tone and form." Literature and the arts, as they relate to medicine, are a learning laboratory **wherein aspirants** to the helping professions enter the lives of the ill where the hurt and anxiety are imaginatively real, to vicariously probe and **ponder** under the **tutelage** of poetry and stories, memoirs and moving pictures. By reading narratives of illness written by gifted writers, physicians can more precisely **fathom** the fears and losses of patients with serious illnesses, identifying in fictional characters and then in their own patients the inevitable conflicts and uncertainties that sickness brings. On the other hand, literary representations of the physician's work, written by nonphysicians as well as physicians, clarify the many roles and expectations of medicine and thereby help readers to understand not only the responsibilities of physicians and the positions of medicine within a culture but also the social crises to which physicians must respond.

In the field of literature, arts, and medicine, we attempt to deal with a series of issues: For example, we will explore why sickness prompts us to storytelling; how popular media influences our views about what it means to grow old or live with a disability, or to practice high-tech hospital medicine; how poetry makes language care; why it's important for doctors to strive to **merge** medical and humanistic sensibilities; and how student-teacher relations affect the moral formation of future health care professionals.

The study of literature contributes in several ways to achievement in the human dimensions of medicine: (1) Literary accounts of illness can teach physicians concrete and powerful lessons about the lives of sick people; (2) great works of fiction about medicine enable physicians to recognize the power and the implications of what they do; (3) through narrative knowledge, physicians can better understand patients' stories of sickness, thereby strengthening diagnostic accuracy and therapeutic effectiveness while deepening an understanding of their own personal **stake** in medical practice; (4) literary study contributes to physicians' expertise in narrative ethics and helps physicians to perform longitudinal acts of ethical **discernment**; and (5) literary theory

---

New Expressions

rendering /'rendərɪŋ/ *n.* 演奏；扮演；表演

wherein /wer'ɪn/ *adv.* 其中；在那里；在那种情况下

aspirant /ə'spaɪərənt/ *n.* 有抱负的人；有雄心壮志的人

ponder /'pɑːndər/ *v.* 沉思；考虑；琢磨

tutelage /'tuːtəlɪdʒ/ *n.* 教导；指导；辅导

fathom /'fæðəm/ *v.* 理解；彻底了解；弄清真相

merge /mɜːrdʒ/ *v.* （使）合并，结合，并入

stake /steɪk/ *n.* 重大利益；重大利害关系

discernment /dɪ'sɜːrnmənt/ *n.* 识别能力；洞察力

offers new perspectives on the work and the genres of medicine. Although our discussion of literature's contributions to medicine focuses on works of fiction, genres, such as poetry, drama, and film are equally valuable to physicians and medical educators.

Notes

1. **Fine arts:** 美术，艺术。在过去，它是指绘画、雕塑、建筑、音乐及诗歌等艺术形式；现在，除了指绘画、雕塑等传统艺术形式外，它还包含摄影、观念艺术等新型艺术形式。"Fine art" is a subjective term that has evolved over time, just as art and artistic styles have evolved. We understand art to be the process of creating something unique that appeals to our visual or auditory senses. Fine art, also referred to as "high art", has long been held up as the highest standard of artistic expression.

2. **liberal arts:** 文理通识。文理通识常用于通识教育（liberal arts education），旨在给学生提供文理通识课程，着重培养学生的理性思维、分析能力和解决问题的能力。它通常包括文学、历史、哲学、经济学、社会学、心理学、生物学、化学、物理学和数学等学科，研究领域涵盖人文科学、社会科学、物理科学和数学等。Liberal arts refer to a broad category of academic disciplines that are traditionally considered essential for a well-rounded education. Liberal arts education emphasizes the development of critical thinking and analytical skills, the ability to solve complex problems, and an understanding of ethics and morality, as well as a desire to continue to learn. Liberal arts colleges provide students with education in both intellectual and practical skills.

3. **John Berger:** 约翰·伯格，1926—2017；英国著名艺术史家、小说家和画家。John Berger, in full John Peter Berger, is a British essayist and cultural thinker as well as a prolific novelist, poet, translator, and screenwriter.

4. **Clifford Geertz:** 利福德·格尔茨，1926—2006；美国人类学家、解释人类学的提出者。格尔茨曾先后担任斯坦福大学行为科学高等研究中心的研究员、加利福尼亚大学巴凯学院人类学系副教授、芝加哥大学新兴国家比较研究会人类学副教授和普林斯顿高等科学研究所社会科学教授。Clifford Geertz is an American cultural anthropologist, a leading rhetorician and proponent of symbolic anthropology and interpretive anthropology.

5. **Cameron:** 卡梅伦，1910—1995；其全名为詹姆斯·蒙罗·卡梅伦（James Munro Cameron）。卡梅伦是加拿大多伦多大学哲学方向荣休教授，著有《大学的理想》

（*On the Idea of a University*）、《夜战》（*The Night Battle*）和《核心天主教徒及其他散文》（*Nuclear Catholics and Other Essays*）等书籍。Cameron is a professor emeritus of philosophy at the University of Toronto. He has published widely and has authored many influential books.

Post-reading Activities

I   Speaking Practice: Group Discussion

Directions: *Please discuss the following questions in small groups. After your discussion, please share your opinions with the whole class.*

1. According to the text, what can physicians gain from reading the narratives of illness and stories of doctoring? Please give examples to illustrate your ideas.

2. According to the text, what are the series of issues that the field of literature, arts, and medicine attempts to deal with?

3. In what ways can the study of literature contribute to achievements in the human dimensions of medicine?

4. Think of a film or a piece of literary work involving aging, death, and pain. What insights have you gained about life and death from appreciating it?

II   Speaking Practice: Oral Presentation

Directions: *Besides medical knowledge, literature and arts are also believed to be indispensable parts of medical students' education. Please give an oral presentation on the importance of the teaching of literature and arts in medical students' education by searching relevant information from different sources.*

Part 2　Thematic Reading

Indian Camp①

At the lake shore there was another **rowboat** drawn up. The two Indians stood waiting.

Nick and his father got in the **stern** of the boat and the Indians **shoved** it off and one of them got in to **row**. Uncle George sat in the stern of the camp rowboat. The young Indian shoved the camp boat off and got in to row Uncle George.

The two boats **started off** in the dark. Nick heard the **oarlocks** of the other boat quite a way ahead of them in the **mist**. The Indians rowed with quick **choppy strokes**. Nick lay back with his father's arm around him. It was cold on the water. The Indian who was rowing them was working very hard, but the other boat moved farther ahead in the mist all the time.

"Where are we going, Dad?" Nick asked.

"Over to the Indian camp. There is an Indian lady very sick."

"Oh," said Nick.

Across the bay they found the other boat **beached**. Uncle George was smoking a cigar in the dark. The young Indian pulled the boat way up the beach. Uncle George gave both the Indians cigars.

New Expressions	
rowboat /ˈroʊboʊt/ *n.* 划艇	**oarlock** /ˈɔːrlɑːk/ *n.*（固定在小船边缘的）桨架
stern /stɜːrn/ *n.* 船尾	**mist** /mɪst/ *n.* 薄雾；水汽
shove /ʃʌv/ *v.* 猛推；乱挤；推撞	**choppy** /ˈtʃɑːpi/ *adj.* 波浪起伏的；不平静的
row /roʊ/ *v.* 划（船）	**stroke** /stroʊk/ *n.* 划水动作；划桨动作
start off 开始活动；动身	**beach** /biːtʃ/ *v.*（使）上岸；把……拖上岸

---

① The text is adapted from the following source: Hemingway, E. 2001. The Indian camp. In R. Reynolds & J. Stone (Eds.), *On Doctoring*. New York: Simon & Schuster, 102–105.

They walked up from the beach through a **meadow** that was **soaking** wet with **dew**, following the young Indian who carried a **lantern**. Then they went into the woods and followed a **trail** that led to the **logging** road that ran back into the hills. It was much lighter on the logging road as the **timber** was cut away on both sides. The young Indian stopped and blew out his lantern and they all walked on along the road.

They came around a **bend** and a dog came out barking. Ahead were the lights of the **shanties** where the Indian **barkpeelers** lived. More dogs rushed out at them. The two Indians sent them back to the shanties. In the **shanty** nearest the road there was a light in the window. An old woman stood in the doorway holding a lamp.

Inside on a wooden **bunk** lay a young Indian woman. She had been trying to have her baby for two days. All the old women in the camp had been helping her. The men had moved off up the road to sit in the dark and smoke **out of range of** the noise she made. She screamed just as Nick and the two Indians followed his father and Uncle George into the shanty. She lay in the lower bunk, very big under a **quilt**. Her head was turned to one side. In the upper bunk was her husband. He had cut his foot very badly with an **ax** three days before. He was smoking a **pipe**. The room smelled very bad.

Nick's father ordered some water to be put on the stove, and while it was heating he spoke to Nick.

"This lady is going to have a baby, Nick," he said.

"I know," said Nick.

"You don't know," said his father. "Listen to me. What she is going through is called being **in labor**. The baby wants to be born and she wants it to be born. All her muscles are trying to get the baby born. That is what is happening when she screams."

New Expressions	
meadow /'medoʊ/ *n.* 草地；牧场	**barkpeeler** /bɑːrk'piːlər/ *n.* 剥树皮的人
soak /soʊk/ *v.* 浸泡；浸湿；浸透；湿透	**bunk** /bʌŋk/ *n.* （尤指儿童的）双层床；架子床；上铺；下铺
dew /duː/ *n.* 露；露水	
lantern /'læntərn/ *n.* 灯笼；提灯	**out of range of** 超出……的范围；在视觉（或听觉）范围之外
trail /treɪl/ *n.* （乡间的）小路，小径	**quilt** /kwɪlt/ *n.* 加衬芯床罩；被子
log /lɑːg/ *v.* 采伐（森林的）树木；伐木	**ax** /æks/ *n.* 斧头
timber /'tɪmbər/ *n.* （建筑等用的）木材，木料	**pipe** /paɪp/ *n.* 烟斗；烟袋
bend /bend/ *n.* （尤指道路或河流的）拐弯，弯道	**in labor** 分娩；生产
shanty /'ʃænti/ *n.* 简陋的小屋；棚屋	

"I see," Nick said.

Just then the woman cried out.

"Oh Daddy, can't you give her something to make her stop screaming?" asked Nick.

"No. I haven't any anesthetic," his father said. "But her screams are not important. I don't hear them because they are not important."

The husband in the upper bunk rolled over against the wall.

The woman in the kitchen **motioned** to the doctor that the water was hot. Nick's father went into the kitchen and poured about half of the water out of the big **kettle** into a **basin**. Into the water left in the kettle he put several things he **unwrapped** from a handkerchief.

"Those must boil," he said, and began to **scrub** his hands in the basin of hot water with a cake of soap he had brought from the camp. Nick watched his father's hands scrubbing each other with the soap. While his father washed his hands very carefully and thoroughly, he talked.

"You see, Nick, babies are supposed to be born head first but sometimes they're not. When they're not they make a lot of trouble for everybody. Maybe I'll have to operate on this lady. We'll know in a little while."

When he was satisfied with his hands he went in and went to work.

"Pull back that quilt, will you, George?" he said. "I'd rather not touch it."

Later when he started to operate, Uncle George and three Indian men held the woman still. She bit Uncle George on the arm and Uncle George said, "Damn **squaw** bitch!" and the young Indian who had rowed Uncle George over laughed at him. Nick held the basin for his father. It all took a long time.

His father picked the baby up and **slapped** it to make it breathe and handed it to the old woman.

New Expressions	
motion /'moʊʃn/ v.（以头或手）做动作，示意	**scrub** /skrʌb/ v. 擦洗；刷洗
kettle /'ketl/ n.（烧水用的）壶，水壶	**squaw** /skwɔː/ n.（旧时用法，常含冒犯之意）
basin /'beɪsn/ n. 盆	美洲印第安女人
unwrap /ʌn'ræp/ v. 打开，解开，拆开（包装）	**slap** /slæp/ v.（用手掌）打，拍，捆

"See, it's a boy, Nick," he said. "How do you like being an **intern**?"

Nick said, "All right." He was looking away so as not to see what his father was doing.

"There. That gets it," said his father and put something into the basin.

Nick didn't look at it.

"Now," his father said, "there's some **stitches** to put in. You can watch this or not, Nick, just as you like. I'm going to sew up the **incision** I made."

Nick did not watch. His curiosity had been gone for a long time.

His father finished and stood up. Uncle George and the three Indian men stood up. Nick put the basin out in the kitchen.

Uncle George looked at his arm. The young Indian smiled **reminiscently**.

"I'll put some **peroxide** on that, George," the doctor said.

He bent over the Indian woman. She was quiet now and her eyes were closed. She looked very pale. She did not know what had become of the baby or anything.

"I'll be back in the morning," the doctor said, standing up. "The nurse should be here from St. Ignace by noon and she'll bring everything we need."

He was feeling **exalted** and talkative as football players are in the dressing room after a game.

"That's one for the medical journal, George," he said. "Doing a **caesarian** with a **jackknife** and sewing it up with nine-foot, **tapered gut leaders**."

Uncle George was standing against the wall, looking at his arm.

"Oh, you're a great man, all right," he said.

New Expressions	
intern /'ɪntɜːrn/ *n.* 实习医生	**exalted** /ɪɡ'zɔːltɪd/ *adj.* 兴奋的；兴高采烈的
stitch /stɪtʃ/ *n.* （缝合伤口的）缝线	**caesarian** /sɪ'zerɪən/ *n.* 剖宫产，剖腹产（手术）
incision /ɪn'sɪʒn/ *n.* 割口；（尤指手术的）切口；切开	**jackknife** /'dʒæknaɪf/ *n.* 大折刀
reminiscently /ˌremɪ'nɪsntli/ *adv.* 回忆过去地；怀旧地；缅怀往事地	**tapered** /'teɪpərd/ *adj.* 锥形的
	gut /ɡʌt/ *n.* 肠道
peroxide /pə'rɑːksaɪd/ *n.* 过氧化物；过氧化氢；双氧水	**tapered gut leader** 渐细的肠线

"Ought to have a look at the proud father. They're usually the worst sufferers in these little affairs," the doctor said. "I must say he took it all pretty quietly."

He pulled back the blanket from the Indian's head. His hand came away wet. He mounted on the edge of the lower bunk with the lamp in one hand and looked in. The Indian lay with his face toward the wall. His throat had been cut from ear to ear. The blood had flowed down into a pool where the bunk **sagged** under the weight of his body. His head rested on his left arm. The **open razor** lay, edge up, in the blankets.

"Take Nick out of the shanty, George," the doctor said.

There was no need of that. Nick standing in the door of the kitchen, had a good view of the upper bunk when his father, the lamp in one hand, **tipped** the Indian's head back.

It was just beginning to be daylight when they walked along the logging road back toward the lake.

"I'm terribly sorry I brought you along, Nickie," said his father, all his **postoperative exhilaration** gone. "It was an awful mess to put you through."

"Do ladies always have such a hard time having babies?" Nick asked.

"No, that was very, very exceptional."

"Why did he kill himself, Daddy?"

"I don't know, Nick. He couldn't stand things, I guess."

"Do many men kill themselves, Daddy?"

"Not very many, Nick."

"Do many women?"

"Hardly ever."

"Don't they ever?"

"Oh, yes. They do sometimes."

New Expressions	
sag /sæg/ *v.* （由于承重或受压）下凹	**tip** /tɪp/ *v.* （使）倾斜，倾倒，翻覆
razor /ˈreɪzər/ *n.* 剃须刀；刮脸刀	**postoperative** /ˌpoʊstˈɑːpərətɪv/ *adj.* 手术后的
open razor　开放式剃须刀	**exhilaration** /ɪɡˌzɪləˈreɪʃn/ *n.* 高兴；兴奋；激动

"Daddy?"

"Yes."

"Where did Uncle George go?"

"He'll turn up all right."

"Is dying hard, Daddy?"

"No, I think it's pretty easy, Nick. It all depends."

They were seated in the boat, Nick in the stern, his father rowing. The sun was coming up over the hills. A **bass** jumped, making a circle in the water. Nick trailed his hand in the water. It felt warm in the sharp chill of the morning.

In the early morning on the lake sitting in the stern of the boat with his father rowing, he felt quite sure that he would never die.

New Expression

bass /bæs/ *n.* 鲈（包括多种食用海鱼和淡水鱼）

Note

Indian Camp: 《印第安人营地》。《印第安人营地》选自欧内斯特·海明威（Ernest Hemingway）的短篇小说集《我们的时代》(*In Our Time*)。在《我们的时代》中，海明威按时间顺序讲述了主人公尼克·亚当斯（Nick Adams）从童年、青少年到壮年的故事。书中用了很大篇幅描述主人公尼克的性格特点。海明威出生于美国伊利诺伊州芝加哥市郊区奥克帕克，美国作家、记者，被认为是20世纪最著名的小说家之一。"Indian Camp" was first published in 1924 in Hemingway's first American volume of short stories *In Our Time*. Ernest Hemingway is an American novelist and short-story writer, who was awarded the Nobel Prize for Literature in 1954. He was noted both for the intense masculinity of his writing and for his adventurous and widely publicized life. His succinct and lucid prose style exerted a powerful influence on American and British fiction in the 20th century.

Post-reading Activities

I Language Building-up

Task 1 Extensive Vocabulary Enlargement

Directions: *The following words are taken from the text. Please follow the three-step learning in this part and build up your own Extensive Vocabulary Chart.*

Step 1. Read through the words and underline them in the text. Circle the ones that are particularly new to you. Look up the words in the dictionary and put the equivalent Chinese translation in the chart below.

Step 2. While you go back to the text, please feel free to put any other words into the blanks provided in the extra lines in the chart.

Extensive Vocabulary Chart				
stern	shove	row	mist	stroke
beach	meadow	lantern	trail	timber
quilt	ax	kettle	intern	caesarian

Step 3. Please group the above words based on their parts of speech and meanings.

Nouns	
Verbs	
Adjectives	

Adverbs and Prepositions	
Medical Terminology	
Terminology in Other Fields	

Task 2 Intensive Vocabulary Enhancement

Directions: *The following 10 words are chosen from the text. They will form the intensive vocabulary in this unit. For intensive vocabulary, you are supposed to be able to explain them in English and use them in sentence and discourse constructions.*

Step 1. Please read through the words and be familiar with their Chinese and English definitions. Recall where and how they are used in the text.

Intensive Vocabulary Chart				
No.	Word	Translation	Definition	Status
1	soak	浸泡；浸湿；浸透；湿透	*v.* to put sth. in liquid for a time so that it becomes completely wet; to become completely wet in this way	☆ ☆ ☆ ☆ ☆
2	unwrap	打开，解开，拆开（包装）	*v.* to take off the paper, etc. that covers or protects sth.	☆ ☆ ☆ ☆ ☆
3	slap	（用手掌）打，拍，掴	*v.* to hit sb./sth. with the flat part of the hand	☆ ☆ ☆ ☆ ☆
4	stitch	（缝合伤口的）缝线	*n.* a short piece of thread, etc. that doctors use to sew the edges of a wound together	☆ ☆ ☆ ☆ ☆
5	incision	割口；（尤指手术的）切口；切开	*n.* a sharp cut made in sth., particularly during a medical operation; the act of making a cut in sth.	☆ ☆ ☆ ☆ ☆
6	reminiscently	回忆过去地；怀旧地；缅怀往事地	*adv.* showing that sb. is thinking about the past, especially in a way that causes him/her pleasure	☆ ☆ ☆ ☆ ☆

Intensive Vocabulary Chart				
No.	Word	Translation	Definition	Status
7	exalted	兴奋的；兴高采烈的	*adj.* full of great joy and happiness	☆ ☆ ☆ ☆ ☆
8	tip	（使）倾斜，倾倒，翻覆	*v.* to move so that one end or side is higher than the other; to move sth. into this position	☆ ☆ ☆ ☆ ☆
9	postoperative	手术后的	*adj.* connected with the period after a medical operation	☆ ☆ ☆ ☆ ☆
10	exhilaration	高兴；兴奋；激动	*n.* a feeling of excitement, happiness, or elation	☆ ☆ ☆ ☆ ☆

Step 2. Please tick the status for each word based on your own situation. If one word is very new or difficult for you, please tick five stars. Likewise, if one word is comparatively easy for you and you don't have to spend too much time on reading and learning it, then tick one star. The number of stars represents the difficulty of commanding a word in your eyes.

Step 3. Please complete the following 10 sentences by choosing appropriate words from the Intensive Vocabulary Chart. Please change the forms of the words where necessary.

1. The mother _____ water into the cup for her child.

2. The surgeon made a small _____ below the patient's rib.

3. The _____ young lady showed her trophy proudly to her friends.

4. He _____ his face into the water to calm himself down.

5. The little girl _____ the cover of the box swiftly to see what's in it.

6. The party is filled with vigor and _____.

7. As compared with open surgery, micro-invasive surgery has less blood loss and shorter _____ hospital stay.

8. The man was terribly hurt and the cut needed at least ten _____.

9. The young man _____ himself in the face due to remorse.

10. The group of old friends talked and smiled _____ in their reunion.

Directions: *The following sentences are taken from the text. In each sentence, there is one phrase being underlined. Please refer to the dictionary and write down the explanation of the phrase in the line entitled "Meaning Exploration". After that, please make a sentence with it. Write the sentence in the line entitled "Sentence Making".*

Sentence 1

Original Sentence	The young Indian stopped and blew out his lantern...
Meaning Exploration	*blow out:*
Sentence Making	

Sentence 2

Original Sentence	The men had moved off up the road to sit in the dark and smoke out of range of the noise she made.
Meaning Exploration	*out of range of:*
Sentence Making	

Sentence 3

Original Sentence	Later when he started to operate, Uncle George and three Indian men held the woman still.
Meaning Exploration	*hold (sb.) still:*
Sentence Making	

Sentence 4

Original Sentence	He pulled back the blanket from the Indian's head.
Meaning Exploration	*pull back:*

Sentence Making	

Sentence 5

Original Sentence	He <u>mounted on</u> the edge of the lower bunk with the lamp in one hand and looked in.
Meaning Exploration	*mount on:*
Sentence Making	

II Critical Reading and Thinking

Task 1 Overview and Comprehension

Directions: *The text is a story written from the perspective of a son narrating one of his doctor father's visits to an Indian patient's family. Please follow the storyline and write down the main information provided in each part based on your reading.*

Reading Notes	
Description of the Patient and Her Husband	
The Whole Process of the Operation Including the Preparation	
The Attitudes of the Son, the Father and the Husband Toward the Woman's Agony	

Task 2 Reflection and Discussion

Directions: *After reading, please reflect on the theme of the text. Work in groups and share your opinions on the following questions with other group members.*

1. Why do you think the father took his son with him when he was going out to see the patients?

2. What did the father mean when he said "But her screams are not important. I don't hear them because they are not important"?

3. What role did Uncle George play in the story?

4. Why did the husband kill himself?

5. What do you think the boy had learned during his father's house call to the Indian camp?

医学人文英语教程

Part 3 Extended Reading

The Doctor Writer: Richard Selzer①1

Richard Selzer's stories **are peopled with** the ill and injured, damaged survivors of close calls, and casualties of the surgical theater. But for all their suffering, these patients are not **pitiable**. They are **estimable**. What is endlessly fascinating to this doctor writer is the sacredness that **pervades** and envelops the space of suffering that they occupy. For Selzer, surgery is a sacred art, **redolent** with ritual. Surgery is sacred not in a **sectarian**, but rather a spiritual sense. Acknowledging "a strong **note** of spirituality" in his work, Selzer remarks, "This is only natural for a writer who sees flesh as the spirit thickened."

Selzer's surgeon is expertly knowledgeable and highly accomplished technically. Beyond these necessary **attributes** of competence, his work is informed and **enlivened** by a certain sensibility, the refined responsiveness to **pathos**. This surgeon has attended many a patient over the years. There was Joe Riker, the short-order cook with a cancer that had eaten a hole through his **scalp** and **skull**, who refused surgery and healed himself with holy water from **Lourdes**2. And Pete, the hospital mailman with **acute abdominal** pain: "**Narcotized**, he nods and takes my fingers in his own, pressing. Thus has he given me all of his trust... 'Go to sleep, Pete,' I say into his ear, my lips so close

New Expressions	
be peopled with　挤满了（人）	**attribute** /'ætrɪbjuːt/ *n.* 属性；性质；特征
pitiable /'pɪtɪəbl/ *adj.* 值得同情的；可怜的	**enliven** /ɪn'laɪvn/ *v.* 使更有生气（或活力）
estimable /'estɪməbl/ *adj.* 值得尊重的；值得敬佩的	**pathos** /'peɪθɑːs/ *n.*（文章、讲话和戏剧的）感染力；令人产生悲悯共鸣的力量
pervade /pər'veɪd/ *v.* 渗透；弥漫；遍及	**scalp** /skælp/ *n.* 头皮
redolent /'redələnt/ *adj.* 使人想到的；使人联想起的	**skull** /skʌl/ *n.* 颅骨；头（盖）骨
sectarian /sek'terɪən/ *adj.*（宗教）教派的	**acute** /ə'kjuːt/ *adj.*（疾病）急性的，严重的
note /noʊt/ *n.* 特征	**abdominal** /æb'dɑːmɪnl/ *adj.* 腹部的
	narcotize /'nɑːrkə,taɪz/ *v.* 麻醉

---

① The text is adapted from the following source: Cole, R. T. et al. 2015. *Medical Humanities: An Introduction.* New York: Cambridge University Press.

it is almost a kiss"—the trust received. Another of Selzer's characters is a young man, back from an excavation of ancient **Guatemalan ruins**[3], who presented himself with an abscessed wound in his upper arm out of which emerged a menacing-looking gray worm with black pincers. With deftness (and even greater self-satisfaction), the surgeon stood poised, hemostat at the ready, and extracted the offender, only to learn from the pathologist that the organism was the larva of a botfly that was burrowing its way out, whereupon it would have dropped to the ground and died without the dramatic intervention of the surgeon. These patients have taught the surgeon humility in the face of the inexplicable, the necessity of fellow feeling and the boon of comfort, and modesty.

Selzer, the writer, is a parabolist. A parable is a story with meaning beyond the literal. This second meaning is not buried beneath the words of the story to be excavated and analyzed, but is there in plain view although only obliquely discernible—perceptible at a slant. Selzer's story, "A Parable", opens with a doctor discreetly witnessing an early morning scene in a hospital room where a man lies, inert and near death, breathing erratically in rapid bursts followed by the suspension of breathing, then more rapid bursts. "It is called **Cheyne-Stokes respiration**[4]. When they start that, you know it won't be long."

An elderly physician in surgical scrubs, stooped and seemingly somewhat worn

New Expressions	
excavation /ˌekskə'veɪʃn/ *n.* 发掘现场	**inexplicable** /ˌɪnɪk'splɪkəbl/ *adj.* 费解的；无法解释的
abscessed /'æbsest/ *adj.* 脓肿的	**boon** /buːn/ *n.* 非常有用的东西；益处
menacing /'menəsɪŋ/ *adj.* 威胁的；恐吓的；危险的	**parabolist** /pə'ræbləst/ *n.* 寓言家
pincer /'pɪnsər/ *n.* 钳子	**parable** /'pærəbl/ *n.* （尤指《圣经》中的）寓言故事
deftness /'deftnəs/ *n.* 熟练；灵巧；机敏	**literal** /'lɪtərəl/ *adj.* 字面意义的
poised /pɔɪzd/ *adj.* 处于准备状态的；蓄势待发的	**in plain view** 一目了然；清晰可见
hemostat /'himəˌstæt/ *n.* 止血器	**obliquely** /ə'bliːkli/ *adv.* 间接地；不直截了当地；拐弯抹角地
at the ready 随时可用；即可使用	**at a slant** 斜着（这里指侧面描写或推断）
extract /ɪk'strækt/ *v.* （用力）取出，拔出	**discreetly** /dɪ'skriːtli/ *adv.* （言行）谨慎地，慎重地；考虑周到地
pathologist /pə'θɑːlədʒɪst/ *n.* 病理学医生；病理学家	**inert** /ɪ'nɜːrt/ *adj.* 无活动能力的；无行动力的
larva /'lɑːrvə/ *n.* 幼虫	**erratically** /ɪ'rætɪkli/ *adv.* 不规则地；不稳定地
botfly /'bɑːtˌflaɪ/ *n.* 肤蝇（类）；狂蝇	**suspension** /sə'spenʃn/ *n.* 暂缓；推迟；延期；（呼吸）暂停
burrow /'bɜːrou/ *v.* 挖掘（洞或洞穴通道）；挖洞	**scrub** /skrʌb/ *n.* 手术衣（常用复数）
whereupon /ˌwerə'pɑːn/ *conj.* 然后；于是；随之；据此；因此	**stoop** /stuːp/ *v.* 俯身；弯腰

down, enters the room. With a **moistened** tissue, he wipes **pus** from around the man's eyes and says something to him that the witness cannot hear. The patient then twice tries to speak but cannot. "When the doctor turns his head to bend an ear to the lips of his patient, I can see the deep **furrow** that divides his brow, extending from the bridge of the nose almost to the hairline. It gives his face a pained expression. It is a line of pain. Had he been born with it? No, I think he had not. Rather, it had appeared on the day that he treated his first patient. At first, it was merely a shadow on his forehead, then a slight **indentation** that, over the years, has deepened into this dark **cleft** that is the mark of all the suffering he has witnessed over a lifetime as a doctor. It **resembles** a wound that might have been made with an ax."

As he **palpates** the patient's abdomen, the doctor asks, "Am I hurting you?" whereupon the patient shakes his head and, astonishingly, stretches a trembling hand toward the doctor's head. "The sick man finds the furrow with his finger, touches, and then **strokes** it from one end to the other, a look of wonder upon his face, as though he were just waking from a deep sleep. As he does so, a **spicule** of light appears to **emanate** from the doctor's forehead. It is a warm light that grows to **engulf** the two men and the bed. From this touching, the doctor does not withdraw, but smiles down at the patient with his **sapphiric** gaze... From the doorway, the two men appear to be luminous... It is as if I were witnessing a **feast**... The two men are dining together, each the **nourishment** of the other." The doctor returns the following morning to find the man lying perfectly still. After unsuccessfully trying to find a pulse, he observes the man's body before placing a hand over his heart and closing his eyes. "As he leaves the room, it seems the furrow is not quite so deep and dark as on the day before."

W. II. Auden[5] said, "You cannot tell people what to do, you can only tell them parables; and that is what art really is, particular stories of particular people and experiences, from which each according to his immediate and peculiar needs may

New Expressions	
moisten /ˈmɔɪsn/ *v.* （使）变得潮湿，变得湿润	**stroke** /strəʊk/ *v.* 轻抚，抚摩（物体表面或头发等）
pus /pʌs/ *n.* 脓	**spicule** /ˈspɪˌkjul/ *n.* 针状物
furrow /ˈfɜːrəʊ/ *n.* （脸上的）皱纹	**emanate** /ˈeməneɪt/ *v.* 产生；表现；显示
indentation /ˌɪndenˈteɪʃn/ *n.* 凹陷；凹痕；缺口	**engulf** /ɪnˈgʌlf/ *v.* 包围；吞没；淹没
cleft /kleft/ *n.* （自然的）裂口，裂缝	**sapphiric** /səˈfɪrɪk/ *adj.* 蓝宝石的
resemble /rɪˈzembl/ *v.* 看起来像；显得像；像	**feast** /fiːst/ *n.* 盛宴；宴会
palpate /pælˈpeɪt/ *v.* 触诊；触摸检查	**nourishment** /ˈnɜːrɪʃmənt/ *n.* 营养；营养品

draw his own conclusions." Parables are narratives that **disclose** moral **quandaries** and illuminate spiritual relations. Instead of leading listeners or readers toward a robust conclusion, as was perhaps possible at times when matters of the spirit were less unsettled than they are today, modern parables often simply raise a question for pondering or persuade by **intimation** and indirection. What all parables, ancient and modern, have in common is the impatience with the obvious and a search for significance that come together in moments of insight. Parables have an **arresting** quality that **etches** them in memory. Because they engage imagination, they penetrate deeply into experience. They possess the power to do more than **provoke** curiosity. They arouse something within by calling up what the hearer, or the reader, vaguely senses but now can fully see.

In his essay, "Religion, Poetry, and the 'Dilemma' of the Modern Writer", **David Daiches**[6] observed that literary and religious answers to questions about suffering tend to be responses rather than solutions. "The answers have force and meaning **in virtue of** their poetic expression, of the place they take in the myth or **fable** or situation presented, and of the effectiveness with which they **project** a mood." The projection of a mood does not solve anything, but, if it is persuasive, it may make life more tolerable, more interesting, even. Moreover, if life is made more tolerable by the telling of stories and the artful use of **imagery**, patients and doctors alike may thereby be enabled to return to the daily round in the face of experiences that would otherwise threaten to become unbearable.

New Expressions

disclose /dɪs'kloʊz/ v. 揭露；透露；泄露

quandary /'kwɑːndəri/ n. 困惑；进退两难；困窘

intimation /ˌɪntɪ'meɪʃn/ n. 透露；间接表示；暗示

arresting /ə'restɪŋ/ adj. 引人注意的；很有吸引力的

etch /etʃ/ v. 蚀刻，凿出（玻璃、金属等上的文字或图画）

provoke /prə'voʊk/ v. 激起；引起；引发

in virtue of 凭借；依靠；由于；因为

fable /'feɪbl/ n. 寓言；寓言故事

project /prə'dʒekt/ v. 展现；表现；确立（好印象）

imagery /'ɪmɪdʒəri/ n. 像；画像；照片

Notes

1. Richard Selzer: 里查德·塞尔泽，1928—2016；美国外科医生、作家，当代最著名的医生作家之一。Surgeon and writer Richard Selzer was born in Troy, New York, graduated from Union College in 1948 and received his M.D. from Albany

Medical College in 1953. After completing a surgical internship and residency at Yale University in 1960, Dr. Selzer remained as the assistant clinical professor of surgery until 1985 in addition to maintaining a private practice. Richard Selzer was one of the most prominent American surgeon-authors.

2. **Lourdes:** 卢尔德市。卢尔德市位于法国西南部，接近西班牙边界的波河（Gave de Pau）岸边，是个朝圣城市。朝圣和庆祝活动在朝圣期间及复活节和万圣节期间达到最大规模。盛大的庆祝礼仪、长长的仪式队伍，以及寻求奇迹的病人，使整个城市沉浸在一种神圣的氛围中。Lourdes, a pilgrimage town, is located in southwestern France, southwest of Toulouse. Situated at the foot of the Pyrenees and now on both banks of a torrent, the Gave de Pau, the town and its fortress formed a strategic stronghold in medieval times.

3. **Guatemalan ruins:** 危地马拉废墟。危地马拉是古代印第安人玛雅文化的发祥地之一，现在仍然可见当时留下来的许多金字塔和城市废墟，极为壮观。In the 1830s, the American John Lloyd Stephens first discovered the ruins of the ancient Maya civilization in the tropical jungle of Honduras. Since then, archaeologists from all over the world have found many abandoned Maya ancient city ruins in the jungle of Central America. The ruins of Guatemala are one of them.

4. **Cheyne-Stokes respiration:** 潮式呼吸。潮式呼吸的特点是呼吸逐步减弱以至停止和呼吸逐渐增强两者交替出现，周而复始，呼吸呈潮水涨落样，其多见于中枢神经疾病、脑循环障碍和中毒等患者。潮式呼吸周期可长达 30 秒~2 分钟，暂停期可持续 5~30 秒。Cheyne-Stokes respiration is a specific form of periodic breathing (waxing and waning amplitude of flow or tidal volume) characterized by a crescendo-decrescendo pattern of respiration between central apneas or central hypopneas.

5. **W. H. Auden:** W. H. 奥登，1907—1973；其全名为威斯坦·休·奥登（Wystan Hugh Auden），著名诗人，被公认为是自 T. S. 艾略特（T. S. Eliot）之后最重要的英语诗人。1968 年，奥登获得诺贝尔文学奖提名。Auden is a famous English poet and was nominated for Nobel Prize in Literature in 1968.

6. **David Daiches:** 戴维·达契斯，1912—2005；英国著名学者、文学批评家。David Daiches is a world-famous English scholar and literary critic.

Post-reading Activities

I Speaking Practice: Role Play

Directions: *Please work in pairs. Read through the part in which the author describes Selzer's story, "A Parable", carefully. Imagine one of you is the doctor described in the story and the other is the patient. Please design a conversation between the doctor and the patient during which they interact with each other. Be sure to use verbal and nonverbal languages to show the patient's suffering and fear as well as the doctor's care and understanding to the patient. Please take turns to be the doctor and the patient.*

Verbal language:

1. _____
2. _____
3. _____

Nonverbal language:

1. _____
2. _____
3. _____

II Reflective Writing Practice: Short Essay

Directions: *Richard Selzer is a famous doctor writer, who wrote a lot of essays based on his experiences as a surgeon. His writing can be viewed both as a mirror reflecting the daily practices among medical professionals and as a bridge connecting the world of doctors' and that of patients'. Please think about the roles doctor writers play in our society and write a reflective essay entitled "The Value of Doctor Writers". Please use concrete examples to illustrate your ideas. The word limit is suggested to be 150–200 words.*

医学人文英语教程

Unit 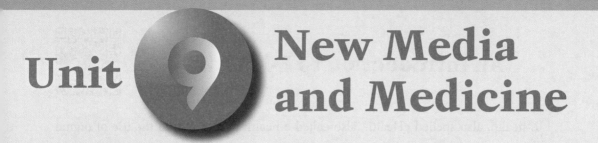 9 New Media and Medicine

We believe consumer health technologies—apps, wearables, self-diagnosis tools—have the potential to strengthen the patient-physician connection and improve health outcomes.
—Glen Stream

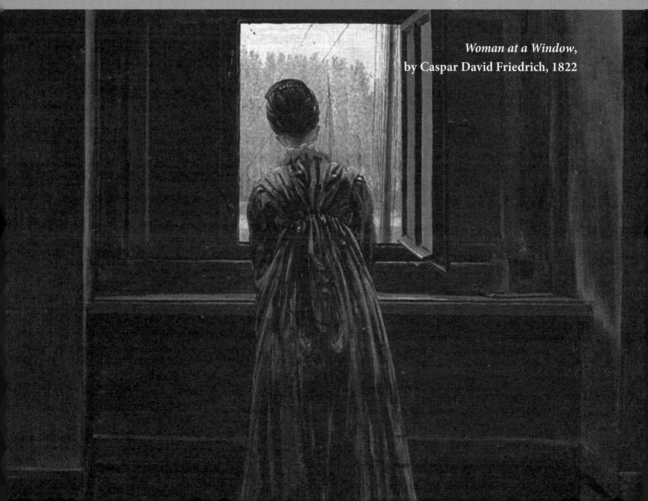

Woman at a Window,
by Caspar David Friedrich, 1822

Part 1 Academic Horizon

An Introduction to E-health[①]

    E-health, also spelled eHealth, also called e-health care, refers to the use of digital technologies and **telecommunications**, such as computers, the Internet, and mobile devices, to facilitate health improvement and health care services. E-health is often used alongside traditional "off-line" (non-digital) approaches for the delivery of information directed to the patient and the health care consumer.

The Need for E-health

    E-health grew out of a need for improved **documentation** and **tracking** of patients' health and procedures performed on patients, particularly for **reimbursement** purposes, such as by **insurance** companies. Traditionally, health care providers kept paper records on the history and status of their patients. However, rising health care costs and technological advances encouraged the development of electronic tracking systems. As e-health technologies continued to be developed, the field of **telemedicine**, in which telecommunication technologies are used to provide health care **remotely**, emerged.

E-health Technologies

    E-health makes use of a wide **array** of digital technologies. The Internet, for example, allows e-health users to communicate with health care professionals by e-mail,

New Expressions	
telecommunication /ˌtelikəˌmjuːnɪˈkeɪʃn/ *n.* 电信	偿；报销
documentation /ˌdɑːkjʊmenˈteɪʃn/ *n.* 文档记载；文献记录；归档	**insurance** /ɪnˈʃʊrəns/ *n.* 保险
tracking /ˈtrækɪŋ/ *n.* 追踪；跟踪	**telemedicine** /ˈtelɪˌmedɪsɪn/ *n.* 远程医疗
reimbursement /ˌriːɪmˈbɜːrsmənt/ *n.* 偿还；补	**remotely** /rɪˈməʊtli/ *adv.* 远程地
	array /əˈreɪ/ *n.* 大堆；大群；大量

---

① The text is adapted from the following source: Peters, K. E. & Glasser, M. L. 2013. E-health. *Encyclopedia Britannica*. Retrieved March 24, 2023, from Encyclopedia Britannica website.

 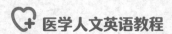 医学人文英语教程

to access medical records, to research health information, and to engage in person-to-person exchange of text, audio, video, and other data. Interactive TV, also known as polycom[1], provides both audio and visual transfer of a variety of information between two or more individuals at two or more locations in real time. Kiosks[2], which are freestanding devices (usually computers), are used in e-health to provide interactive information to the user. Most information is provided through a series of interactive prompts on a touch screen. Kiosks can also be used to collect data and information from users. DVDs, USB flash drives, and other media are used to store data digitally. Many modern mobile devices are designed with personal computing and Internet capabilities and are compatible with downloadable applications (or apps) that allow users to instantly access health information. Many of the technologies employed in e-health are accessible to all users, including those with impairments, such as blindness or deafness.

Benefits and Barriers

There are benefits and barriers to both providers and consumers who use e-health. Beneficial impacts include the use by physicians of computerized drug-ordering systems that can reduce the risk of adverse drug events[3] through decision support systems. Similarly, automated computerized reminders can increase orders for recommended prevention interventions, such as yearly physicals, mammograms, and prostate examinations. In more extreme situations, e-health has been used by emergency medical personnel and first responders[4] for consultation during natural disasters and in military battlefield situations. In rural and remote areas this technology has been used by primary care providers to provide consultations for patients through direct linkage to urban-based specialists. E-health has also been used as a distance education strategy

New Expressions	
access /'ækses/ v. 访问；获取	be compatible with 适合；与……一致；与……兼容
engage in 从事；参加	
audio /'ɔːdiou/ n. 音频	computerized /kəm'pjuːtəraɪzd/ adj. 电脑化的
interactive /ˌɪntər'æktɪv/ adj. 交互式的；人机对话的；互动的	automated /'ɔːtəmeɪtɪd/ adj. 自动化的
	physical /'fɪzɪkl/ n. 体检；体格检查
freestanding /ˌfriː'stændɪŋ/ adj. 单独的；独立的	mammogram /'mæməgræm/ n. 乳房 X 光检查
prompt /prɑːmpt/ n. 提示符	prostate /'prɑːsteɪt/ n. 前列腺
flash drive 闪存盘	consultation /ˌkɑːnsl'teɪʃn/ n. 咨询；商讨；磋商
computing /kəm'pjuːtɪŋ/ n. 信息处理技术	distance education 远程教育

for primary and continuing education. **International collaborative initiatives** have benefited from advances in e-health by making information readily available to health care professionals and consumers.

Consumer benefits from advances in e-health include, for example, the ability to order prescriptions over the Internet for direct delivery to the home. Hospitals and other **acute care** institutions host web pages that detail their expertise and services for patients. E-health has also benefited persons with disabilities who **reside** in the community by permitting provider-patient communication through text, audio, or **video conferencing** to **gauge** home-based progress.

Barriers to the use of e-health by health care providers include a lack of financial **incentives** and a lack of reimbursement to support its use within and across organizations. In addition, the initial **incorporation** of new e-health technologies often slows established processes (due to the **learning curve** needed to implement new tools and devices) before the more **streamlined** system is established. Other barriers to e-health technologies include costs, such as those associated with hardware and software purchases and **maintenance** and upgrades, and the lack of standards concerning the format and content of e-health information, particularly private patient health-related information, which has legal and economic implications for providers with regard to **liability** and **malpractice** insurance.

One of the largest barriers to widespread consumer use of e-health is the so-called **digital divide**. The digital divide can be defined as a disparity in access to digital technologies, particularly the Internet. Whereas people on one side of the divide have access to those technologies and possess the knowledge needed to use them, people on the other side of the divide typically do not. Although access to electronic

New Expressions	
international collaborative initiative 国际合作倡议	**learning curve** 学习曲线
acute care 紧急护理	**streamlined** /'striːmlaɪnd/ *adj.* 效率更高的
reside /rɪ'zaɪd/ *v.* 居住在；定居于	**maintenance** /'meɪntənəns/ *n.* 维护；保养
video conferencing 视频会议	**liability** /ˌlaɪə'bɪləti/ *n.*（法律上应承担的）责任，义务
gauge /geɪdʒ/ *v.* 判定；判断；测量	**malpractice** /ˌmæl'præktɪs/ *n.* 渎职；玩忽职守
incentive /ɪn'sentɪv/ *n.* 激励；刺激；鼓励	**digital divide** 数字鸿沟
incorporation /ɪnˌkɔːrpə'reɪʃn/ *n.* 吸收；纳入	

communications is **steadily** increasing in both developed and less-developed countries, the increases are not uniform, and disparities in availability and skill levels persist. Issues, such as costs, **literacy** levels, cultural **appropriateness**, and compliance with standards for those with disabilities (e.g. **Americans with Disabilities Act**[5] of 1990) are significant barriers in the use of e-health. Other issues include those associated with the protection of privacy and confidentiality and informed consent, as well as those related to the ease of e-health technologies.

New Expressions	
steadily /'stedəli/ *adv.* 稳定地	**appropriateness** /ə'prəupriətnəs/ *n.* 恰当性；合适性
literacy /'lɪtərəsi/ *n.* 读写能力	

Notes

1. **polycom:** 宝利通（文中指代交互式电视）。观众可以利用电子设备选择不同的观赏角度以获得最佳视觉效果或与电视节目中的人物进行对话。Polycom is the integration of traditional television technology and data services. It is a two-way cable system that allows users to interact with it via commands and feedback information.

2. **Kiosks:** 自助服务机，信息服务亭。自助服务机是提供产品或储存信息及提供媒体展示的自助式服务设备。该类设备整合了各式软硬件设备，以影片、图片、文字、音乐等多媒体数据库形成的互动环境，提供各类产品贩卖或信息服务。Kiosk is a small stand-alone device providing information and services on a computer screen.

3. **adverse drug events:** 药品不良事件。药品不良事件是指患者使用药品出现的任何不利的医学事件，且不一定与此治疗存在因果关系。不良事件可以是与使用药品有时间关联的、任何不利的且与用药目的无关的体征（如异常实验室结果）、症状或疾病，无论其是否与该药品有因果关系。An adverse drug event is an injury resulting from medical intervention related to a drug. This includes medication errors, adverse drug reactions, allergic reactions, and overdoses.

4. **first responders:** 第一急救者。第一急救者是指受过专业培训、第一时间到达现场处理紧急情况的人，包括警察、消防员、医疗人员等。A first responder is a person who is trained to respond to an emergency situation. The term can refer to a wide range of professionals, including police officers, firefighters, and paramedics.

5. Americans with Disabilities Act:《美国残疾人法案》。这是一项具有里程碑意义的立法，其主要目的是保护残疾人免受歧视，减少或消除残疾人在日常生活中面临的许多障碍，该法案于 1990 年由美国国会通过并由布什总统签署。The Americans with Disabilities Act (ADA) is a federal civil rights law that prohibits discrimination against people with disabilities in everyday activities. The ADA prohibits discrimination on the basis of disability just as other civil rights laws prohibit discrimination on the basis of race, color, sex, national origin, age, and religion.

Post-reading Activities

I Speaking Practice: Group Discussion

Directions: *Please discuss the following questions in small groups. After your discussion, please share your opinions with the whole class.*

1. What ideas would come to your mind when you hear the term "e-health"?
2. Have you used any e-health technologies in your everyday or professional life?
3. What are the benefits of e-health from your own perspective?

II Speaking Practice: Oral Presentation

Directions: *In the last paragraph of the text, "digital divide" is highlighted as "one of the largest barriers to widespread consumer use of e-health". Please search for information about digital divide in health care on the Internet and then give an oral presentation to introduce the issue to the whole class.*

Part 2 Thematic Reading

The Doctor, the Patient, and the World Wide Web: How the Internet Is Changing Health Care[①]

The Internet is increasingly being employed for health information and health care delivery. Clinicians need to understand the possibilities of this technology, and to be aware of potential threats to health.

The Internet as a Resource for Health Information

One of the main uses of the Internet is as an encyclopedic information resource. Surveys consistently show that 60%–80% of World Wide Web users have used it to obtain health information. The Internet has the potential to educate and empower the health consumer, by providing information on health and health services and supporting self-help and patient choice. Two-thirds of those using the Internet to find health information claim it has some impact on their health care decisions.

Many concerns have been raised about the quality of online consumer health information, and the possibility that poor information has detrimental effects on health. Online health information is often incomplete and sometimes inaccurate. While there have been isolated case reports of individuals coming to harm from information on the Internet, there is no systematic evidence that more harm arises from this medium than

New Expressions	
encyclopedic /ɪnˌsaɪkləˈpiːdɪk/ adj. 百科全书的；百科知识的	incomplete /ˌɪnkəmˈpliːt/ adj. 不完整的；不完善的
survey /ˈsɜːrveɪ/ n. 民意调查；民意测验	inaccurate /ɪnˈækjərət/ adj. 不精确的；不准确的；有错误的
detrimental /ˌdetrɪˈmentl/ adj. 有害的；不利的	

---

① The text is adapted from the following source: Powell, J. A. et al. 2003. The doctor, the patient and the World Wide Web: How the Internet is changing health care. *Journal of the Royal Society of Medicine*, 96(2): 74–76.

from others. Education of consumers or content producers may help reduce the spread of poor information.

The Internet also supports professional health information. Clinicians are benefiting from increased access to evidence, policy and guidelines, and training and professional development. Health **datasets**, increasingly available online, will facilitate research.

The Internet as a Medium for Interaction

It is the **interactivity** of the Internet that possibly has the most profound impact on health and health care. The universal and **pervasive** e-mail is making fundamental changes to the way that people work. E-mail communication between doctors and patients is becoming part of medical practice—although a U.S. survey suggests that doctors are **reluctant** to embrace this new medium until they are convinced it will save time or money.

The revolution in communication and knowledge exchange between individuals is most evident in the phenomenon of **virtual** communities. In the health area, an example is the support for people with HIV. **Peer to peer support** in virtual communities benefits from the absence of traditional barriers to access; and online **anonymity** can be helpful for those who have stigmatizing or **embarrassing** conditions. The international possibilities of virtual communities allow individuals with **rare diseases** to find peer support and allow all users to draw on a wide range of health perspectives and experience. However, there are concerns that the lack of professional moderation or facilitation in most virtual communities may lead to inappropriate and **disruptive** use, or to the **dissemination** of inaccurate messages.

New Expressions

dataset /'deɪtəset/ *n.* 数据集

interactivity /ˌɪntəræk'tɪvəti/ *n.* 互动性

pervasive /pər'veɪsɪv/ *adj.* 遍布的；充斥各处的；弥漫的

reluctant /rɪ'lʌktənt/ *adj.* 不情愿的；勉强的

virtual /'vɜːrtʃuəl/ *adj.* （通过计算机软件，如在互联网上）仿真的，虚拟的

peer to peer support 同伴互助

anonymity /ˌænə'nɪməti/ *n.* 匿名；不知姓名；名字不公开

embarrassing /ɪm'bærəsɪŋ/ *adj.* 使人害羞的（或难堪的、惭愧的）

rare disease 罕见病

disruptive /dɪs'rʌptɪv/ *adj.* 引起混乱的；扰乱性的；破坏性的

dissemination /dɪˌsemɪ'neɪʃn/ *n.* 散布，传播（信息、知识等）

The Internet as a Tool for the Delivery of Health Care

The Internet is increasingly being used for health care delivery. Health promotion and education interventions have been successfully delivered online, and there are early reports of psychological interventions via the Internet. A study showed that an e-mail discussion group had a positive effect on health status in people with chronic back pain. **Specialties** which have used telemedicine for remote diagnosis and **asynchronous** communication can now explore the enhanced possibilities of the Internet—for example to provide "virtual **outreach**" consultations in areas with poor access to conventional services.

The development of **electronic patient records**[1] and the networking of **primary and secondary care**[2] have the potential to improve the quality and efficiency of health services. The Internet can also be used as a medium for health research—using online interviews, **focus groups**[3], and **quantitative** survey methods.

Shifting the Balance of Power

The Internet is changing the balance of knowledge between health care professionals and the public, empowering patients to become more involved in health care decision-making and contributing to the **deprofessionalization of medicine**[4]. The professional power of medicine is being challenged by the public availability of specialist knowledge, and by improved access to information on alternative approaches to health care, health care performance **statistics**, and consumer rights.

Many patients now bring Internet printouts to the consultation, and benefits to patients are being reported. However, "Internet printout **syndrome**" or "**cyberchondria**[5]" has generally been **portrayed** as a time-consuming affliction of the "worried well". The Internet offers the potential for patients to become more involved in their own care, learning about their condition, accessing and contributing to their online health record,

New Expressions
specialty /'speʃəlti/ n. 专业；专长
asynchronous /eɪ'sɪŋkrənəs/ adj. 不同时存在（或发生）的；非共时的
outreach /'aʊtriːtʃ/ n. 外展服务（在服务机构以外的场所提供的社区服务等）
quantitative /'kwɑːntəteɪtɪv/ adj. 量化的；定量的
statistic /stə'tɪstɪk/ n. 统计数据
syndrome /'sɪndrəʊm/ n. 综合征；综合症状
portray /pɔːr'treɪ/ v. 将……描写成；给人以某种印象；表现

and interacting with health services—for example using **shared decision-making**[6] tools. Clinicians can assist by recommending high-quality websites and listing these in information sheets.

The Internet and Public Health

The advent of an Internet-enabled "information society" could have much broader consequences. For example, network access is supporting more home working, which could impact on public health in many ways: Decreased individual travel and increased commercial deliveries of goods may reduce traffic pollution and accidents, but may also reduce social interaction and physical exercise. Effects are to be expected on home life, productivity, and energy consumption. At present, the Internet is predominantly a computer-mediated tool, and there is a need to quantify its health impact with respect to ergonomic issues—for example, postural musculoskeletal disorders.

The Internet allows development of communities—explicit in chatroom formats, but also implicit communities of individuals linking with each other through hypertext or e-mail connections. In this way, the Internet can support campaigning and democratization, giving users the means to organize socially and politically, and it can facilitate the working of communities of practice (such as public health networks).

Access Issues: The Have-nets and the Have-nots

The term "digital divide" has been coined to describe the gaps in access and understanding that may exclude certain groups from use of new digital technologies. As one might expect, the groups most at risk of digital exclusion are those that already have unequal access to health services and suffer health inequalities—for example, the poor, the homeless, those with limited formal education, disabled or elderly people, and those in developing countries.

New Expressions	
predominantly /prɪˈdɑːmɪnəntli/ adv. 主要地；多数情况下	**musculoskeletal** /ˌmʌskjəloʊˈskelətl/ adj. 肌（与）骨骼的
computer-mediated /kəmˈpjuːtər ˈmiːdieɪtɪd/ adj. 以计算机为媒介的	**explicit** /ɪkˈsplɪsɪt/ adj. 清楚明白的；易于理解的
ergonomic /ˌɜːrɡəˈnɑːmɪk/ adj. 工效学的；人类工程学的	**hypertext** /ˈhaɪpərtekst/ n. 超文本
postural /ˈpɑːstʃərəl/ adj.（坐、立）姿势的	**democratization** /dɪˌmɑːkrətəˈzeɪʃn/ n. 民主化
	exclude /ɪkˈskluːd/ v. 不包括；不放在考虑之列
	at risk of 冒……的危险

医学人文英语教程

The Internet offers the possibility of reducing inequalities in health—through low-cost dissemination of consumer and professional information, remote delivery of health services, and **removal** of barriers to access. But care must be taken to ensure that differential access to new technology does not **exacerbate** existing inequalities in health. The World Health Organization has expressed concern at the digital divide between the developed and developing worlds and this has led to initiatives, such as the **Health Internetwork**[7] which aims to provide free access to resources, such as biomedical publications.

Conclusions

The Internet is having profound impacts on health and health care. It has the potential to improve the effective and efficient delivery of health care, empower and educate consumers, support decision-making, enable interaction between consumers and professionals, support the training and **revalidation** of professionals, and reduce inequalities in health. But there is a need for **vigilance** regarding new and emerging threats to health posed by the Internet. Investigation of both positive and negative health impacts of this **evolving** technology must continue. Work in this area must acknowledge the importance of the wider determinants of health: In addition to the more obvious direct effects, the impact of the Internet on domains, such as the economy, employment, environment, and transport will all influence health and health care.

New Expressions	
removal /rɪ'muːvl/ *n.* 除去；消除；清除	**revalidation** /riːˌvælɪ'deɪʃn/ *n.* 再认证
exacerbate /ɪg'zæsərbeɪt/ *v.* 使恶化；使加剧；使加重	**vigilance** /'vɪdʒɪləns/ *n.* 警觉；警惕；警戒
	evolving /ɪ'vɑːlvɪŋ/ *adj.* 发展变化中的

Notes

1. **electronic patient records**: 电子病历。电子病历是指医务人员在医疗活动过程中，使用信息系统生成的文字、符号、图表、图形、数字、影像等数字化信息，并能实现存储、管理、传输和重现的医疗记录，是病历的一种记录形式，包括门（急）诊病历和住院病历。An electronic patient record is an electronic version of a patient's medical history, which is maintained by the provider over time, and may include all of the key administrative clinical data relevant to that person's care

under a particular provider, including demographics, progress notes, problems, medications, vital signs, past medical history, immunizations, laboratory data and radiology reports.

2. **primary and secondary care:** 初级和二级医疗。初级医疗指一般的医疗保健，即病人在转诊到医院或专科前的一些医疗。二级医疗指专科医生及医院所提供的部分服务。Primary care is the first level of care that patients receive and is focused on patient wellness, prevention of health conditions and management of a chronic disease. Secondary care refers to all the medical services patients will receive after they've had their primary care doctors see them.

3. **focus groups:** 焦点小组，也称小组访谈。焦点小组是社会科学研究中常用的质性研究方法，一般由一个经过研究训练的调查者主持，采用半结构方式（即预先设定部分访谈问题的方式）与一组被调查者交谈。其主要目的是倾听被调查者对研究问题的看法。A focus group refers to a demographically diverse group of people assembled to participate in a guided discussion about a particular issue, or to provide ongoing feedback on a political campaign, television series, etc.

4. **deprofessionalization of medicine:** 医学去专业化。随着医学知识的公开和普及，以及医疗方案获取方式的多样化，医学的专业力量正受到挑战，这种现象被称为医学去专业化。The professional power of medicine is being challenged by the public availability of specialist knowledge, and by improved access to information on alternative approaches to health care, health care performance statistics, and consumer rights. This phenomenon is referred to as deprofessionalization of medicine.

5. **cyberchondria:** 网络疑病症。网络疑病症是指查看了网络上的症状描述后想象自己也患上了同样的疾病。Cyberchondria refers to a clinical phenomenon in which repeated Internet searches regarding medical information result in excessive concerns about physical health.

6. **shared decision-making:** 共同决策。共同决策是一个过程，涉及医生和患者充分了解医疗检测和治疗的好处、风险及效果，确定病人偏好和优先事项，并达成共识，制定诊疗方案。Shared decision-making is a process that involves patients and clinicians in understanding the benefits, harms, and effectiveness of health care tests and treatments; determining personal priorities and values; and mutually agreeing upon a course of action.

7. **Health Internetwork:** 卫生互联网（网站名称）。卫生互联网是由联合国秘书长发起、世界卫生组织领导的旨在跨越健康领域"数字鸿沟"的项目，目的是推动卫生信息与技术的广泛传播与利用。The Health Internetwork was established in 2002. The team comprises a panel of experts, who specialize in their field of knowledge, touching on topics, such as health, fitness, and relationships. The website strives to deliver comprehensive, unbiased reviews along with valuable information to its readers.

Post-reading Activities

I Language Building-up

Task 1 Extensive Vocabulary Enlargement

Directions: *The following words are taken from the text. Please follow the three-step learning in this part and build up your own Extensive Vocabulary Chart.*

Step 1. Read through the words and underline them in the text. Circle the ones that are particularly new to you. Look up the words in the dictionary and put the equivalent Chinese translation in the chart below.

Step 2. While you go back to the text, please feel free to put any other words into the blanks provided in the extra lines in the chart.

Extensive Vocabulary Chart				
encyclopedic	survey	detrimental	inaccurate	interactivity
anonymity	disruptive	dissemination	specialty	asynchronous
outreach	quantitative	statistic	syndrome	ergonomic
postural	hypertext	democratization	revalidation	evolving

Step 3. Please group the words on the previous page based on their parts of speech and meanings.

Nouns	
Verbs	
Adjectives	
Adverbs and Prepositions	
Medical Terminology	
Terminology in Other Fields	

Task 2　Intensive Vocabulary Enhancement

Directions: *The following 10 words are chosen from the text. They will form the intensive vocabulary in this unit. For intensive vocabulary, you are supposed to be able to explain them in English and use them in sentence and discourse constructions.*

Step 1. Please read through the words and be familiar with their Chinese and English definitions. Recall where and how they are used in the text.

Intensive Vocabulary Chart				
No.	Word	Translation	Definition	Status
1	pervasive	遍布的；充斥各处的；弥漫的	*adj.* existing in all parts of a place or thing; spreading gradually to affect all parts of a place or thing	☆ ☆ ☆ ☆ ☆

Intensive Vocabulary Chart				
No.	Word	Translation	Definition	Status
2	reluctant	不情愿的；勉强的	*adj.* hesitating before doing sth. because sb. does not want to do it or because sb. is not sure that it is the right thing to do	☆ ☆ ☆ ☆ ☆
3	virtual	（通过计算机软件，如在互联网上）仿真的，虚拟的	*adj.* made to appear to exist by the use of computer software, for example on the Internet	☆ ☆ ☆ ☆ ☆
4	portray	将……描写成；给人以某种印象；表现	*v.* to describe or show sb./sth. in a particular way, especially when this does not give a complete or accurate impression of what it is like	☆ ☆ ☆ ☆ ☆
5	predominantly	主要地；多数情况下	*adv.* mostly; mainly	☆ ☆ ☆ ☆ ☆
6	explicit	清楚明白的；易于理解的	*adj.* (of a statement or piece of writing) clear and easy to understand	☆ ☆ ☆ ☆ ☆
7	exclude	不包括；不放在考虑之列	*v.* to deliberately not include sth. in what sb. is doing or considering	☆ ☆ ☆ ☆ ☆
8	removal	除去；消除；清除	*n.* the act of getting rid of sth.	☆ ☆ ☆ ☆ ☆
9	exacerbate	使恶化；使加剧；使加重	*v.* to make sth. worse, especially a disease or problem	☆ ☆ ☆ ☆ ☆
10	vigilance	警觉；警惕；警戒	*n.* the process of paying close and continuous attention	☆ ☆ ☆ ☆ ☆

Step 2. Please tick the status for each word based on your own situation. If one word is very new or difficult for you, please tick five stars. Likewise, if one word is comparatively easy for you and you don't have to spend too much time on reading and learning it, then tick one star. The number of stars represents the difficulty of commanding a word in your eyes.

Step 3. Please complete the following 10 sentences by choosing appropriate words from the Intensive Vocabulary Chart. Please change the forms of the words where necessary.

1. The reasons for the decision should be made _____.

2. The symptoms may be _____ by certain drugs.

3. She stressed the need for constant _____.

4. She was _____ to admit she was wrong.

5. A sense of social change is _____ in her novels.

6. _____ of the benign tumor is not necessary in such cases.

7. She works in a(n) _____ male environment.

8. New technology has enabled development of an online "_____ library".

9. Throughout the trial, he _____ himself as the victim.

10. Some of the data was specifically _____ from the report.

Task 3 Expressions and Sentences

Directions: *The following sentences are taken from the text. In each sentence, there are one or two phrases being underlined. Please refer to the dictionary and write down the explanation of the phrases in the line entitled "Meaning Exploration". After that, please choose one phrase and make a sentence with it. Write the sentence in the line entitled "Sentence Making".*

Sentence 1

Original Sentence	The Internet has the potential to educate and empower the health consumer, by providing information on health and health services and supporting self-help and patient choice.
Meaning Exploration	*have the potential to:*
Sentence Making	

Sentence 2

Original Sentence	Two-thirds of those using the Internet to find health information claim it has some impact on their health care decisions.
Meaning Exploration	*have (an) impact on:*
Sentence Making	

Sentence 3

Original Sentence	E-mail communication between doctors and patients is becoming part of medical practice—although a U.S. survey suggests that doctors are reluctant to embrace this new medium until they are convinced it will save time or money.
Meaning Exploration	*be reluctant to*: *be convinced (that)*:
Sentence Making	

Sentence 4

Original Sentence	The term "digital divide" has been coined to describe the gaps in access and understanding that may exclude certain groups from use of new digital technologies.
Meaning Exploration	*exclude (sb./sth.) from*:
Sentence Making	

Sentence 5

Original Sentence	As one might expect, the groups most at risk of digital exclusion are those that already have unequal access to health services and suffer health inequalities—for example, the poor, the homeless, those with limited formal education, disabled or elderly people, and those in developing countries.
Meaning Exploration	*at risk of*:
Sentence Making	

II Critical Reading and Thinking

Task 1 Overview and Comprehension

Directions: *The text could be divided into eight parts. Please write down the main information provided in each part based on your reading.*

Reading Notes	
Introduction	
The Internet as a Resource for Health Information	
The Internet as a Medium for Interaction	
The Internet as a Tool for the Delivery of Health Care	
Shifting the Balance of Power	
The Internet and Public Health	
Access Issues: The Have-nets and the Have-nots	
Conclusions	

Task 2　Reflection and Discussion

Directions: *After reading, please reflect on the theme of the text. Work in groups and share your opinions on the following questions with other group members.*

1. Online health information may be inaccurate or even misleading. As a health consumer, what can you do to distinguish between reliable and unreliable sources of information?

2. What are the benefits and drawbacks of communicating in online health communities?

医学人文英语教程

3. Telemedicine and online medical consultations have become part of contemporary health care. What are the main challenges doctors and patients face when communicating on the Internet?

4. How does the Internet shift the balance of power between medical professionals and the lay public?

5. In what ways does the Internet help reduce health inequalities?

Part 3 Extended Reading

Social Media and Medicine[①]

The way we communicate in the 21st century has transformed with the advent of social media. Social media use is pervasive, and its reach has been **leveraged** extensively outside of medicine, helping marketing and promotion. In the clinical field, patients are both actively seeking medical knowledge on social media and exposed to health-related content through these platforms. Therefore, active engagement by clinicians on social media where health knowledge is sought presents an opportunity for **patient education**[1] and **humanization** of the medical profession.

Over the years, a number of social media platforms have emerged, including Facebook, Twitter, Instagram, YouTube and TikTok, all of which have been adapted for mobile devices. Today, patients, health professionals, major medical journals, government agencies, hospitals, and academic institutions actively contribute to online discourse on social media. Conversely, certain individuals, groups, and organizations continue to disseminate **unsubstantiated** health claims and **endorsements** of non-evidence-based ideas and products. Although the subject of online misinformation over social media is highly complex, some have suggested the need for more trained professionals to serve as sources of accurate health information and cite literature as a misinformation **countermeasure**.

In medical training, marketing **tactics** and social media training is not typically

New Expressions	
leverage /ˈlevərɪdʒ/ v. 充分利用	**endorsement** /ɪnˈdɔːrsmənt/ n.（公开的）赞同，支持，认可
humanization /ˌhjuːmənəˈzeɪʃn/ n. 人性化；人本化；人类化	**countermeasure** /ˈkaʊntərmeʒər/ n. 对策；对抗手段；反措施
unsubstantiated /ˌʌnsəbˈstænʃieɪtɪd/ adj. 未经证实的；未被证明的	**tactic** /ˈtæktɪk/ n. 策略；手段；招数

---

① The text is adapted from the following source: Chiang, A. L. 2020. Social media and medicine. *Nature Reviews Gastroenterology & Hepatology*, 17(5): 256–257.

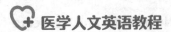 医学人文英语教程

considered part of a standard curriculum. As a result, not only do physicians lack the training to effectively cultivate a presence on social media, but there is little guidance currently on its responsible execution. Given increasing distrust of medical professionals by the general public, it is therefore paramount that further guidance be developed to help health professionals utilize social media in an effective and responsible manner. Within health care, varying formats and a multitude of features enable each social media platform to serve different purposes and inform different audiences. Some professionals choose to utilize social media for educational purposes, whereas others focus on self-expression, advocacy, or development of other non-clinical business efforts. Regardless of one's purpose on social media, health professionals must uphold professional standards and abide by institutional policies or risk disciplinary action or jeopardize public trust in the medical profession.

With over an estimated 3.5 billion individuals worldwide, nearly half the global population actively uses social media. In addition to standard text and video-based content, many of these platforms contain additional features, such as group chat rooms, live streaming, audience polling, and short-form videos[2] to further help creators engage with their audience. Major platforms, such as Facebook and YouTube boast over 2 billion monthly active users. Twitter, often regarded as the premier forum for academic and professional discourse, commands over 330 million monthly active users worldwide. With brevity as its most notable quality, Twitter limits each post to 280-characters and, therefore, encourages rapid dissemination of concise information.

Social media benefits medical professional users in numerous ways. First, social media facilitates accelerated consumption of health information through the direct distribution of news and publications by society and journal accounts, as well as through

New Expressions	
curriculum /kə'rɪkjələm/ *n.* （学校等的）全部课程	及；危害；损害
execution /ˌeksɪ'kjuːʃn/ *n.* 实行；执行；实施	**live streaming**　现场直播
distrust /dɪs'trʌst/ *n.* 不信任；怀疑	**polling** /'pəʊlɪŋ/ *n.* 投票
paramount /'pærəmaʊnt/ *adj.* 至为重要的；首要的	**boast** /bəʊst/ *v.* 有（值得自豪的东西）
abide by　遵守，遵循（法律、协议、协定等）	**premier** /prɪ'mɪr/ *adj.* 首要的；最著名的；最成功的；第一的
disciplinary action　纪律处分	**brevity** /'brevəti/ *n.* 简洁；简练
jeopardize /'dʒepərdaɪz/ *v.* 冒……的危险；危	**accelerated** /ək'seləreɪtɪd/ *adj.* 加速的；加快的

online discussion with peers including structured online chats and journal clubs. Second, developing professional relationships with colleagues and **thought leaders**[3] internationally within one's profession has never been easier across geographical borders and time zones. Beyond cultivating a valuable network, productive discussions online can reveal clinical challenges that could lead to collaboration in research or other **joint ventures** that advance public health. Third, **health education**[4] on social media could influence public health by improving **health literacy**, **dispelling** misconceptions about the medical profession and directly **debunking** misinformation from inaccurate sources. Likewise, under appropriate protocols, the reach of social media has been used in patient **recruitment** for **clinical trials**. Last, physician presence on social media has been associated with boosting institutional reputation.

Conversely, there are a multitude of potential **pitfalls** of health professional social media use that could ultimately lead to professional consequences and affect public opinions and health. First, protecting patient privacy within the social media environment is not limited only to avoiding standard identifiers, such as likeness and name, but also in reference to descriptions of specific **scenarios** or procedures, timing of posts relative to procedures that are performed, and dissemination of procedural images or **radiographs**. Second, preserving trust in the medical profession also requires **empathizing** with the patient perspective and respecting the portrayal of both patients and ourselves. One example is how activities portrayed outside the clinical setting can also shape patients' opinions of one's clinical competence as well as influence perception of the medical profession as a whole. Interactions with colleagues and patients alike, both publicly and in private messaging should, therefore, be approached **thoughtfully** as though they are public and permanent. Inappropriate or **inflammatory** behavior could **spark**

New Expressions	
joint venture 合营企业；合资企业	**scenario** /sə'næriou/ *n.* 设想；方案；预测
health literacy 健康素养	**radiograph** /'reɪdɪəʊˌɡrɑːf/ X 光照片
dispel /dɪ'spel/ *v.* 驱散, 消除（尤指感觉或信仰）	**empathize** /'empəθaɪz/ *v.* 有同感；产生共鸣；表同情
debunk /ˌdiː'bʌŋk/ *v.* 批判；驳斥；揭穿……的真相	**thoughtfully** /'θɔːtfəli/ *adv.* 体贴地；关心别人地；关切地
recruitment /rɪ'kruːtmənt/ *n.* 招募	**inflammatory** /ɪn'flæmətɔːri/ *adj.* 煽动性的；使人发怒的
clinical trial 临床试验	**spark** /spɑːrk/ *v.* 引发；触发
pitfall /'pɪtfɔːl/ *n.* 危险；困难；（尤指）陷阱，隐患	

public **backlashes** and could also be further **amplified** on social media. Furthermore, on the subject of communication with patients online, the distinction between medical education and personalized medical advice must be understood. Medical advice should never be delivered over the Internet, as these online encounters should not **substitute** in-person evaluation and are often an incomplete assessment of patients. Often, **solicitations** of medical advice can inspire social media content that is regarded as generalized medical education rather than an individualized assessment. Furthermore, to preserve the integrity of online health information and minimize misinformation, health professionals should consider speaking within one's scope of training, citing only high-quality evidence from **peer-reviewed**[5] medical literature, which might prevent misinformation.

The landscape of social media and health is highly dynamic and constantly evolves with shifting platform policies and the **perpetual** introduction of new features. Although **appraising** the benefits of social media on public health continues to be important, a thoughtful approach to avoiding potential pitfalls and greater exploration into how best to reduce barriers of social media adoption remain vital. The complexity of social media content creation and **navigating** challenges in social media with little **formalized** training highlights the need for more guidance and investigation.

New Expressions

backlash /'bæklæʃ/ n. （对社会变动等的）强烈抵制，集体反对

amplify /'æmplɪfaɪ/ v. 放大，增强（声音等）

substitute /'sʌbstɪtuːt/ v.（以……）代替，取代

solicitation /səˌlɪsɪ'teɪʃn/ n. 索求；请求；征求；筹集

perpetual /pər'petʃuəl/ adj. 持续的；长久的

appraise /ə'preɪz/ v. 估量；估价

navigate /'nævɪɡeɪt/ v. 找到正确方法（对付困难、复杂的情况）

formalize /'fɔːrməlaɪz/ v.（通过规则）使有固定体系，使定形

Notes

1. **patient education:** 患者教育。患者教育是指向患者提供与其病情相关信息的过程，如症状和警示、可行的治疗方案、预期结果和副作用，以及预防指南等。Patient education is the process of providing patients with information relevant to their condition, such as symptoms and warning signs, available treatment plans, expected outcomes and side effects, prevention guidelines, etc.

2. **short-form videos:** 短视频。短视频是一种互联网内容传播方式，一般是指在互联网新媒体上传播时长在 1 分钟以内的视频。A short-form video is any type of video content that is less than 60 seconds. Short-form videos are meant to be bite-sized, easily digestible pieces of content that are easy for viewers to scroll through and view several at a time.

3. **thought leaders:** 思想领袖。思想领袖是指在某一特定领域具有公认权威地位的个人或组织，其创新思想用于影响和指导他人。A thought leader refers to a person or organization that is a recognized authority in a particular field and whose innovative ideas influence and guide others.

4. **health education:** 健康教育。健康教育是为个人或公众设计的一种教育形式，旨在向受众普及与健康相关的知识、技能、价值和态度。Health education is a type of education designed for individuals or the public at large to gain the knowledge, skills, value, and attitudes necessary to promote, maintain, improve, and restore their, or another person's health.

5. **peer-reviewed:** 同行评审的。同行评审是一种审查程序，即一位作者的知识产品让同一领域的其他专家学者来加以评审。Peer review is the process of evaluating submissions to an academic journal. Using strict criteria, a panel of reviewers in the same subject area decides whether to accept each submission for publication.

Post-reading Activities

I Speaking Practice: Interview

Directions: *Please work in pairs. Imagine one of you is an interviewee, a doctor who actively posts patient education videos on social media, and the other is an interviewer who interviews the doctor about his/her experience of using social media to facilitate patient education. Please design three interview questions and take turns to be the interviewer and the interviewee.*

Interview questions:

1. _____

2. _____

3. _____

Ⅱ Reflective Writing Practice: Short Essay

Directions: *Social media is increasingly used by patients, health professionals, and government agencies for various health-related purposes. Please think about the application of social media in the medical setting and write a reflective essay entitled "The Potential and Pitfalls of Social Media Use by Medical Professionals". Please use concrete examples to illustrate your ideas. The word limit is suggested to be 150–200 words.*

Unit 10 Doctor-patient Communication

> *Medicine is an art whose magic and creative ability have long been recognized as residing in the interpersonal aspects of patient-physician relationship.*
> —Judith A. Hall, Debra L. Roter, and Cynthia S. Rand

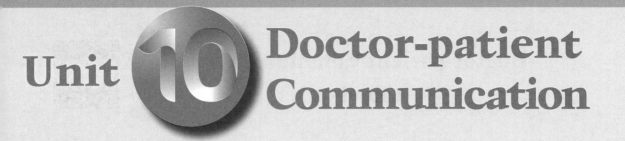

Francisco Goya Self-portrait with Dr. Arrieta,
by Francisco de Goya, 1820

Part 1 Academic Horizon

Doctor-patient Communication: A Review[①]

A doctor's communication and interpersonal skills **encompass** the ability to gather information in order to facilitate accurate diagnosis, counsel the patients appropriately, give therapeutic instructions, and establish caring relationships with patients. These are the **core** clinical skills in the practice of medicine, with the ultimate goal of achieving the best outcome and patient satisfaction, which are essential for the effective delivery of health care.

Basic communication skills in isolation are insufficient to create and **sustain** a successful therapeutic doctor-patient relationship, which consists of shared perceptions and feelings regarding the nature of the problem, goals of treatment, and psychosocial support. Interpersonal skills build on this basic communication skill. Appropriate communication integrates both patient- and doctor-centered approaches.

The ultimate objective of any doctor-patient communication is to improve the patients' health and medical care. Studies on doctor-patient communication have demonstrated patient discontent even when many doctors considered the communication adequate or even excellent. Doctors tend to **overestimate** their abilities in communication. **Tongue**[1] et al. reported that 75% of the **orthopedic** surgeons surveyed believed that they communicated satisfactorily with their patients, but only 21% of the patients reported satisfactory communication with their doctors. Patient surveys have consistently shown that they want better communication with their doctors.

New Expressions	
encompass /ɪnˈkʌmpəs/ *v.* 包含，包括，涉及（大量事物）	**sustain** /səˈsteɪn/ *v.* 使保持；使稳定持续
	overestimate /ˌoʊvərˈestɪmeɪt/ *v.* 高估
core /kɔːr/ *adj.* 最重要的；主要的；基本的	**orthopedic** /ˌɔːrθəˈpiːdɪk/ *adj.* 矫形外科的

---

① The text is adapted from the following source: Ha, J. F. et al. 2010. Doctor-patient communication: A review. *The Ochsner Journal, 10*(1): 38–43.

 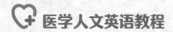

Benefits of Effective Communication

Effective doctor-patient communication is a central clinical function, and the **resultant** communication is the heart and art of medicine and a central component in the delivery of health care. The three main goals of current doctor-patient communication are creating a good interpersonal relationship, facilitating exchange of information, and including patients in decision-making. Effective doctor-patient communication is determined by the doctors' "**bed-side manner**", which patients judge as a major indicator of their doctors' general competence.

Good doctor-patient communication has the potential to help regulate patients' emotions, facilitate comprehension of medical information, and allow for better identification of patients' needs, perceptions, and expectations. Patients reporting good communication with their doctors are more likely to be satisfied with their care, and especially to share **pertinent** information for accurate diagnosis of their problems, follow advice, and **adhere to** the prescribed treatment. Patients' agreement with the doctors about the nature of the treatment and need for follow-up is strongly associated with their recovery.

Studies have shown **correlations** between a sense of control and the ability to **tolerate** pain, recovery from illness, decreased tumor growth, and **daily functioning**. Enhanced psychological adjustments and better mental health have also been reported. Some studies have observed a decrease in the length of **hospital stay** and therefore the cost of individual **medical visits** and fewer referrals. A more **patient-centered encounter** results in better patient as well as doctor satisfaction. Satisfied patients are less likely to **lodge** formal **complaints** or initiate malpractice complaints. Satisfied patients

New Expressions	
resultant /rɪˈzʌltənt/ *adj.* 因而发生的；因此而产生的	**daily functioning**　日常生活功能
	hospital stay　住院时间
bed-side manner　（医护人员等）对待患者的态度	**medical visit**　就医；就诊
	patient-centered encounter　以患者为中心的诊疗
pertinent /ˈpɜːrtnənt/ *adj.* 有关的；恰当的；相宜的	
	lodge /lɑːdʒ/ *v.* （向公共机构或当局）正式提出（声明等）
adhere to　遵守	
correlation /ˌkɔːrəˈleɪʃn/ *n.* 相互关系；相关；关联	**complaint** /kəmˈpleɪnt/ *n.* 投诉；控告；抱怨；埋怨；不满的原因
tolerate /ˈtɑːləreɪt/ *v.* 忍受；容忍；包容	

are **advantageous** for doctors in terms of greater job satisfaction, less work-related stress, and reduced burnout.

The Problems

There are many barriers to good communication in the doctor-patient relationship, including patients' anxiety and fear, doctors' burden of work, fear of **litigation**, fear of physical or verbal **abuse**, and unrealistic patient expectations.

There are also reported observations of doctors avoiding discussion of the emotional and social impact of patients' problems because it **distressed** them when they could not handle these issues or they did not have the time to do so adequately. This situation negatively affected doctors emotionally and tended to increase patients' distress. This **avoidance** behavior may result in patients' being unwilling to disclose problems, which could delay and **adversely** impact their recovery.

Strategies for Improvement

Communication Skills

Communication skills involve both style and content. Attentive listening skills, empathy, and use of open-ended questions are some examples of skillful communication. Improved doctor-patient communication tends to increase patient involvement and **adherence** to recommended therapy; influence patient satisfaction, adherence, and health care utilization; and improve quality of care and health outcomes.

Breaking bad news[2] to patients is a complex and challenging communication task in the practice of medicine. Relationship building is especially important in breaking bad news. Important factors include understanding patients' perspectives, sharing information, and patients' knowledge and expectations. Miscommunication has serious implications, as it may **hinder** patients' understanding, expectations of treatment, or involvement in treatment planning. In addition, miscommunication decreases patients' satisfaction with medical care, level of hopefulness, and subsequent psychological

New Expressions	
advantageous /ˌædvən'teɪdʒəs/ *adj.* 有利的；有好处的	**avoidance** /ə'vɔɪdəns/ *n.* 避免；防止；回避；避开
litigation /ˌlɪtɪ'geɪʃn/ *n.* 诉讼；打官司	**adversely** /əd'vɜrsli/ *adv.* 不利地；有害地；反面地
abuse /ə'bjuːs/ *n.* 虐待	**adherence** /əd'hɪrəns/ *n.* 坚持；遵守；遵循
distress /dɪ'stres/ *v.* 使忧虑；使悲伤；使苦恼	**hinder** /'hɪndər/ *v.* 阻碍；妨碍；阻挡

医学人文英语教程

adjustment. Baile et al. reported that patients often regard their doctors as one of their most important sources of psychological support. Empathy is one of the most powerful ways of providing this support to reduce patients' feelings of isolation and validating their feelings or thoughts as normal and to be expected.

Communication Training

Doctors are not born with excellent communication skills, as they have different innate talents. Instead they can understand the theory of good doctor-patient communication, learn and practice these skills, and be capable of modifying their communication style if there is sufficient motivation and incentive for self-awareness, self-monitoring, and training. Communication skills training has been found to improve doctor-patient communication. However, the improved behaviors may lapse over time. It is therefore important to practice new skills, with regular feedback on the acquired behaviors. Some have said that medical education should go beyond skills training to encourage physicians' responsiveness to the patients' unique experience.

Collaborative Communication

Collaborative communication is a reciprocal and dynamic relationship, involving the two-way exchange of information. In an ideal world, doctors should collaborate with their patients to provide the best care because doctors tend to make decisions based on quick assessments, which may be biased. This requires the doctors to take time or set up opportunities to offer and discuss treatment choices to patients and share the responsibility and control with them. Successful information exchange ensures that concerns are elicited and explored, and that explanations of treatment options are balanced and understood to allow for shared decision-making. In this approach, the doctor facilitates discussion and negotiation with patients and the treatment options are evaluated and tailored to the context of the patients' situation and needs, rather than a standardized protocol. Care options need to be collaborative between doctors and patients, taking into account patient expectations, outcome preferences, levels of

New Expressions	
validate /'vælɪdeɪt/ *v.* 证实；确认；确证	**self-monitoring** /ˌself 'mɑːnɪtərɪŋ/ *n.* 自我监控
innate /ɪ'neɪt/ *adj.* 天生的；先天的；与生俱来的	**lapse** /læps/ *v.* 衰退；衰弱；（逐渐）消失，结束
	reciprocal /rɪ'sɪprəkl/ *adj.* 互惠的；相应的
self-awareness /ˌself ə'wernəs/ *n.* 自我意识	**biased** /'baɪəst/ *adj.* 有偏见的；倾向性的；片面的

risk acceptance, and any associated cost to maximize adherence and to assure the best outcome.

Notes

1. **Tongue:** 唐，1946—2019；其全名为约翰·理查德·唐（John Richard Tongue），医学博士、美国俄勒冈健康与科学大学医学院骨科与康复科临床副教授。Dr. Tongue served as the 80th President of the American Academy of Orthopedic Surgeons in 2012, and as the faculty member at AAHKS Annual Meetings (AAHKS refers to American Association of Hip and Knee Surgeons). He was instrumental in passing the Oregon Safety Belt Law using his first-hand experience in orthopedic trauma and received the 1991 Public Service Award from the National Highway Traffic Safety Association.

2. **Breaking bad news:** 坏消息告知。对医疗工作者来说，对患者或患者家属的坏消息告知通常是个巨大的挑战。在医疗领域，最极端的例子包括关于患者死亡、终末期疾病及残疾等情况的坏消息告知，这些坏消息告知给医生和患者都会带来巨大的精神压力。为减轻双方的压力并达到最佳告知效果，医疗工作者需要学习相关告知技巧，以采用更合适、更专业的方式告知坏消息。Breaking bad news poses great challenges to both medical professionals and patients. Generally, news of death, terminal illness, or deformity constitute the more extreme situations, and will generally be accepted as "bad news" for the recipient. However, news of chronic illnesses or the need for medical intervention, which at first glance would appear less disastrous, could have far-reaching or negative implications for the recipients' personal or working life, or their hopes for the future. No matter in extreme or mild situations, it is always important for medical professionals to deliver bad news in appropriate ways.

Post-reading Activities

I Speaking Practice: Group Discussion

Directions: *Please discuss the following questions in small groups. After your discussion, please share your opinions with the whole class.*

1. According to the text, what are the three main goals of current doctor-patient communication?
2. What are the benefits of effective communication in clinical encounters?
3. What are the barriers to effective doctor-patient communication?
4. What can you do to improve doctor-patient communication?

II Speaking Practice: Oral Presentation

Directions: *From the text, we know that "Breaking bad news to patients is a complex and challenging communication task in the practice of medicine." Please search for information on how to deliver bad news in doctor-patient communication and give an oral presentation on bad news delivery. You may talk about the important role bad news delivery plays in medical encounters and the effective ways to help doctors to deliver bad news to patients. Please give examples to illustrate your ideas.*

Part 2 Thematic Reading

The Use of "Force"[1]

They were new patients to me, all I had was the name, Olson. "Please come down as soon as you can. My daughter is very sick."

When I arrived I was met by the mother, a big **startled** looking woman, very clean and **apologetic** who merely said, "Is this the doctor?" and let me in. In the back, she added. "You must excuse us, doctor. We have her in the kitchen where it is warm. It is very **damp** here sometimes."

The child was fully dressed and sitting on her father's lap near the kitchen table. He tried to get up, but I motioned for him not to bother, took off my overcoat, and started to **look** things **over**. I could see that they were all very nervous, eyeing me up and down distrustfully.

The child was fairly eating me up with her cold, steady eyes, and there was no expression on her face whatever. She did not move and seemed, inwardly, quiet; an unusually attractive little thing, and as strong as a **heifer** in appearance. But her face was **flushed**, she was breathing rapidly, and I realized that she had a high fever. She had **magnificent blonde** hair, in **profusion**.

"She's had a fever for three days," began the father "and we don't know what it comes from. My wife has given her things, you know, like people do, but it didn't work."

New Expressions	
startled /ˈstɑːrtld/ *adj.* 受惊吓的	**flushed** /flʌʃt/ *adj.* 脸红的
apologetic /əˌpɑːləˈdʒetɪk/ *adj.* 道歉的；谢罪的；愧疚的	**magnificent** /mæɡˈnɪfɪsnt/ *adj.* 壮丽的；宏伟的；值得赞扬的
damp /dæmp/ *adj.* 潮湿的；微湿的；湿气重的	**blonde** /blɑːnd/ *adj.*（头发）金黄色的
look... over 查看；检查	**profusion** /prəˈfjuːʒn/ *n.* 大量；众多
heifer /ˈhefər/ *n.*（尤指未生育过的）小母牛	

---

① The text is adapted from the following source: William, C. W. 2001. The use of force. In R. Reynolds & J. Stone (Eds.), *On Doctoring*. New York: Simon & Schuster, 73–76.

 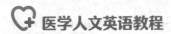

As doctors often do I **took a trial shot** at it as **a point of departure**. "Has she had a **sore** throat?" Both parents answered me together, "No... No, she says her throat doesn't hurt her."

"Does your throat hurt you?" added the mother to the child. But the little girl's expression didn't change nor did she move her eyes from my face.

"Have you looked?" I asked.

"I tried to," said the mother, "but I couldn't see."

"As it happens we had been having a number of cases of **diphtheria**[2] in the school to which this child went during that month and we were all, quite apparently, thinking of that, though no one had as yet spoken of the thing."

"Well," I said, "suppose we take a look at the throat first." I smiled in my best professional manner and asked for the child's first name. I said, "Come on, Mathilda, open your mouth and let's take a look at your throat."

Nothing doing.

"Aw, come on," I **coaxed**, "just open your mouth wide and let me take a look." "Look," I said opening both hands wide, "I haven't anything in my hands. Just open up and let me see."

"Such a nice man," put in the mother, "look how kind he is to you. Come on, do what he tells you to. He won't hurt you."

At that I **ground** my teeth in **disgust**. If only they wouldn't use the word "hurt" I might be able to get somewhere. But I did not allow myself to be hurried or **disturbed** but speaking quietly and slowly I **approached** the child again.

As I moved my chair a little nearer, suddenly with one catlike movement both her hands clawed **instinctively** for my eyes and she almost reached them too. In fact, she

New Expressions	
take a trial shot　　试着做；试探性地发问	disgust /dɪsˈɡʌst/ *n.* 厌恶；憎恶；反感
a point of departure　　出发点；起点	disturb /dɪˈstɜːrb/ *v.* 打扰；干扰；妨碍
sore /sɔːr/ *adj.* （发炎）疼痛的，酸痛的	approach /əˈproʊtʃ/ *v.* （在距离或时间上）靠近，接近
diphtheria /dɪfˈθɪrɪə/ *n.* 白喉	
coax /koʊks/ *v.* 哄劝；劝诱	instinctively /ɪnˈstɪŋktɪvli/ *adv.* 本能地；直觉地；天生地
grind /ɡraɪnd/ *v.* 磨碎；碾碎；把……磨成粉	

knocked my glasses flying and they fell, though unbroken, several feet away from me on the kitchen floor.

"You bad girl," said the mother, taking her and shaking her by one arm. "Look what you've done. The nice man..."

"For heaven's sake," I broke in. "don't call me a nice man to her. I'm here to look at her throat on the chance that she might have diphtheria and possibly die of it." But that's nothing to her. "Look here," I said to the child, "we're going to look at your throat. You're old enough to understand what I'm saying. Will you open it now by yourself or shall we have to open it for you?"

Not a move. Even her expression hadn't changed. Her breaths however were coming faster and faster. Then the battle began. I had to do it. I had to have a **throat culture** for her own protection.

"If you don't do what the doctor says you'll have to go to the hospital." the mother **admonished** her severely.

"Oh yeah?" I had to smile to myself. After all, I had already fallen in love with the **savage brat**. But the parents were **contemptible** to me. In the **ensuing** struggle they grew more and more **abject**, **crushed**, exhausted while she surely rose to magnificent heights of **insane fury** of effort **bred** of her terror of me.

"Put her in front of you on your lap," I ordered, "and hold both her **wrists**."

But as soon as he did the child let out a scream. "You're hurting me! Let go of my hands! Let them go I tell you!" Then she **shrieked terrifyingly**, **hysterically**. "Stop it! Stop it! You're killing me!"

"Do you think she can stand it, doctor!" said the mother.

New Expressions	
throat culture　咽拭子培养	**crushed** /krʌʃt/ *adj.* 被击垮的
admonish /əd'mɑːnɪʃ/ *v.* 责备；告诫；警告	**insane** /ɪn'seɪn/ *adj.* 十分愚蠢的；疯狂的；危险的
savage /'sævɪdʒ/ *adj.* 蒙昧的；未开化的；野蛮的	**fury** /'fjʊrɪ/ *n.* 狂怒；暴怒
brat /bræt/ *n.* 没有规矩的人；（尤指）顽童	**breed** /briːd/ *v.* 孕育；导致
contemptible /kən'temptəbl/ *adj.* 可轻蔑的；可鄙的；卑劣的	**wrist** /rɪst/ *n.* 手腕；腕关节
ensuing /ɪn'ʃʊɪŋ/ *adj.* 接着发生的；因而产生的	**shriek** /ʃriːk/ *v.* 尖叫
abject /'æbdʒekt/ *adj.* 下贱的；卑躬屈节的；自卑的	**terrifyingly** /'terɪfaɪɪŋli/ *adv.* 可怕地；吓人地
	hysterically /hɪ'sterɪkli/ *adv.* 歇斯底里地

"You get out," said the husband to his wife. "do you want her to die of diphtheria?"

"Come on now; hold her." I said.

Then I grasped the child's head with my left hand and tried to get the wooden tongue **depressor** between her teeth. She fought, with **clenched** teeth, desperately! But now I also had grown **furious,** at a child. I tried to hold myself down but I couldn't. I know how to expose a throat for **inspection.** And I did my best. When finally I got the wooden **spatula** behind the last teeth and just the point of it into the mouth **cavity,** she opened up for an instant but before I could see anything she came down again and gripping the wooden **blade** between her **molars**[3] she reduced it to **splinters** before I could get it out again.

"Aren't you ashamed," the mother yelled at her, "aren't you ashamed to act like that in front of the doctor?"

"Get me a smooth-handled spoon of some sort," I told the mother, "we're going through with this." The child's mouth was already bleeding. Her tongue was cut and she was screaming in wild hysterical shrieks. But the worst of it was that I too had **got beyond reason.** I could have **torn** the child apart in my own fury and enjoyed it. It was a pleasure to attack her. My face was burning with it.

In a final unreasoning **assault** I **overpowered** the child's neck and jaws. I forced the heavy silver spoon back of her teeth and down her throat till she **gagged.** And there it was—both **tonsils** covered with **membrane.** She had fought **valiantly** to keep me from knowing her secret. She had been hiding that sore throat for three days at least and lying to her parents in order to escape just such an outcome as this.

New Expressions	
depressor /dɪ'presər/ *n.* 压舌板	**get beyond reason** 失去理智
clench /klentʃ/ *v.* 咬紧（牙齿等）	**tear** /ter/ *v.* 撕裂；撕破；扯破；戳破
furious /'fjʊrɪəs/ *adj.* 狂怒的；暴怒的	**assault** /ə'sɔːlt/ *n.* 攻击；突击；袭击
inspection /ɪn'spekʃn/ *n.* 检查；查看；审视	**overpower** /ˌoʊvər'paʊər/ *v.*（以较强力量）征服，制胜
spatula /'spætʃələ/ *n.* 压舌板	
cavity /'kævəti/ *n.* 洞；孔；窟窿；腔	**gag** /ɡæɡ/ *v.* 作呕
blade /bleɪd/ *n.* 刀身；刀片；刀刃；（文中指）压舌板	**tonsil** /'tɑːnsl/ *n.* 扁桃体
molar /'moʊlər/ *n.* 磨牙；臼齿	**membrane** /'membreɪn/ *n.*（身体内的）膜
splinter /'splɪntər/ *n.*（木头、金属、玻璃等的）尖碎片，尖细条	**valiantly** /'vælɪəntli/ *adv.* 英勇地；勇敢地；果敢地；坚定地

Now truly she was furious. She had been on the defensive before but now she attacked. Tried to get off her father's lap and fly at me while tears of defeat blinded her eyes.

Notes

1. **The Use of "Force":**《使用"暴力"》。本文作者威廉·卡洛斯·威廉斯（William Carlos Williams，1883—1963）是 20 世纪美国最负盛名的诗人之一，与象征派和意象派联系紧密。除此之外，他还是全科及小儿科医师。William Carlos Williams famously combined the two careers of doctor and writer, along the way founding a specifically American version of modernism.

   本文选自《行医之道》（*On Doctoring*）一书。本书由理查德·雷诺兹（Richard Reynolds）等编辑出版，到目前为止共出版三版，时间分别是 1991 年、1995 年和 2001 年。本书汇集了医生和其他作家记录和撰写的关于生老病死的故事、诗歌和短文，记录了医学的广度与奇迹，以及医生和患者在面临各种挑战时所迸发出的发人深省的精神与力量。In this era of managed health care, when medicine is becoming more institutionalized and impersonal, this book recaptures the breadth and the wonder of the medical profession. Presenting the issues, concerns, and challenges facing doctors and patients alike, *On Doctoring* is at once illuminating and provocative, a compelling record of the human spirit.

2. **diphtheria:** 白喉。白喉是一种由白喉棒状杆菌菌株引起的严重感染，这种细菌会产生毒素，并可能导致呼吸困难、心律问题，甚至死亡。这种严重的细菌感染通常会对鼻子和喉咙的黏膜产生影响。Diphtheria is a serious infection caused by strains of bacteria called *Corynebacterium diphtheriae* that make toxins. It can lead to difficulty in breathing, heart rhythm problems, and even death.

3. **molars:** 大白齿，简称白齿，俗称磨牙，是人类和其他哺乳动物的一种牙齿。大白齿位于口腔后方，因上端扁平而且主要用来研磨和咀嚼食物而得名。臼齿由于随使用而被磨损，可以被用来判定生物个体或其遗骸的年龄。Molar is the tooth with a rounded or flattened surface adapted for grinding specifically. It's one of the cheek teeth in mammals behind the incisors and canines.

Post-reading Activities

I   Language Building-up

Task 1   Extensive Vocabulary Enlargement

Directions: *The following words are taken from the text. Please follow the three-step learning in this part and build up your own Extensive Vocabulary Chart.*

Step 1. Read through the words and underline them in the text. Circle the ones that are particularly new to you. Look up the words in the dictionary and put the equivalent Chinese translation in the chart below.

Step 2. While you go back to the text, please feel free to put any other words into the blanks provided in the extra lines in the chart.

Extensive Vocabulary Chart				
damp	heifer	flushed	blonde	profusion
diphtheria	coax	grind	disturb	instinctively
culture	savage	abject	insane	hysterically
clench	molar	tonsil	membrane	valiantly

Step 3. Please group the above words based on their parts of speech and meanings.

Nouns	

Verbs	
Adjectives	
Adverbs and Prepositions	
Medical Terminology	
Terminology in Other Fields	

Task 2　Intensive Vocabulary Enhancement

Directions: *The following 10 words are chosen from the text. They will form the intensive vocabulary in this unit. For intensive vocabulary, you are supposed to be able to explain them in English and use them in sentence and discourse constructions.*

Step 1. Please read through the words and be familiar with their Chinese and English definitions. Recall where and how they are used in the text.

Intensive Vocabulary Chart				
No.	Word	Translation	Definition	Status
1	startle	使惊吓；使吓一跳；使大吃一惊	*v.* to surprise sb. suddenly in a way that slightly shocks or frightens him/her	☆ ☆ ☆ ☆ ☆
2	apologetic	道歉的；谢罪的；愧疚的	*adj.* feeling or showing that sb. is sorry for doing sth. wrong or for causing a problem	☆ ☆ ☆ ☆ ☆
3	sore	（发炎）疼痛的，酸痛的	*adj.* painful, and often red, especially because of infection or because a muscle has been used too much	☆ ☆ ☆ ☆ ☆
4	disgust	厌恶；憎恶；反感	*n.* a strong feeling of dislike or disapproval for sb./sth.	☆ ☆ ☆ ☆ ☆

No.	Word	Translation	Definition	Status
		Intensive Vocabulary Chart		
5	approach	（在距离或时间上）靠近，接近	*v.* to move nearer	☆ ☆ ☆ ☆ ☆
6	admonish	责备；告诫；警告	*v.* to tell sb. firmly that you do not approve of sth. that he/she has done	☆ ☆ ☆ ☆ ☆
7	contemptible	可轻蔑的；可鄙的；卑劣的	*adj.* deserving of contempt or scorn	☆ ☆ ☆ ☆ ☆
8	ensuing	接着发生的；因而产生的	*adj.* following immediately and as a result of what went before	☆ ☆ ☆ ☆ ☆
9	crush	破坏，毁坏（某人的信心和幸福）	*v.* to destroy sb.'s confidence or happiness	☆ ☆ ☆ ☆ ☆
10	breed	孕育；导致	*v.* to be the cause of sth.	☆ ☆ ☆ ☆ ☆

Step 2. Please tick the status for each word based on your own situation. If one word is very new or difficult for you, please tick five stars. Likewise, if one word is comparatively easy for you and you don't have to spend too much time on reading and learning it, then tick one star. The number of stars represents the difficulty of commanding a word in your eyes.

Step 3. Please complete the following 10 sentences by choosing appropriate words from the Intensive Vocabulary Chart. Please change the forms of the words where necessary.

1. They were very _____ about the trouble they'd caused.

2. The passengers all scolded the old man for his _____ behavior on the bus.

3. The schoolmaster _____ the student for his breaking the rules again.

4. Ignorance _____ arrogance and prejudice.

5. She felt completely _____ by the teacher's criticism.

6. The plants revived as spring _____.

7. In the _____ game, the young man will meet his old opponent.

8. The smell of the food is _____!

9. The little girl was _____ when she saw a dog rushed out of the door.

10. His teeth are _____ due to inflammation.

Directions: *The following sentences are taken from the text. In each sentence, there are one or two phrases being underlined. Please refer to the dictionary and write down the explanation of the phrases in the line entitled "Meaning Exploration". After that, please choose one phrase and make a sentence with it. Write the sentence in the line entitled "Sentence Making".*

Sentence 1

Original Sentence	... took off my overcoat, and started to look things over.
Meaning Exploration	look (sth.) over:
Sentence Making	

Sentence 2

Original Sentence	As doctors often do I took a trial shot at it as a point of departure.
Meaning Exploration	as a point of departure:
Sentence Making	

Sentence 3

Original Sentence	... we were all, quite apparently, thinking of that, though no one had as yet spoken of the thing.
Meaning Exploration	as yet: speak of:
Sentence Making	

Sentence 4

Original Sentence	... while she surely rose to magnificent heights of insane fury of effort bred of her terror of me.

Meaning Exploration	*rise to*:
	bred of:
Sentence Making	

Sentence 5

Original Sentence	I could have <u>torn</u> the child <u>apart</u> in my own fury and enjoyed it.
Meaning Exploration	*tear (sb./sth.) apart*:
Sentence Making	

II Critical Reading and Thinking

Task 1   Overview and Comprehension

Directions: *The text is a special event encountered by the doctor. In this text, the doctor used "force" on the girl patient to resolve the problem. Please read the text carefully and write down the main information provided in each part.*

Reading Notes	
What Can You Learn About the Parents at the Beginning?	
How Did the Doctor Try to Examine the Throat of the Little Girl?	
How Did the Doctor Feel About the Parents?	

Directions: *After reading, please reflect on the theme of the text. Work in groups and share your opinions on the following questions with other group members.*

1. Why did the author say he had "fallen in love with" the little girl while getting angry with the parents?

2. If you were the doctor, what would you do in this case? Are there any ways to make the little girl less fearful and more cooperative?

3. Please reflect on the process of doctor-patient communication in this story. Is there anything wrong with the way the doctor used to communicate with the patient and her family members?

4. Please reflect on the process of parent-child communication in this story. Is there anything wrong with the way the parents communicated with the child?

Part 3 Extended Reading

Specific Goals and Strategies of Communicating with Patients[①]

Our ultimate goal is to help the patient achieve optimal health status. We know that the better we are at communicating, the better chance we have of achieving that goal.

The patient's perception of us and our communication skills **rests on** what Aristotle described as the "**rhetorical triangle**". This image illustrates how the three components are dependent on each other, ultimately define how our patients perceive us, and perhaps ultimately determine our ability to achieve our clinical goals. If we use an **abrupt** or **off-putting** tone or style, the patient may think we are not **credible** or trustworthy (**ethos**[1]), and the communication triangle **collapses**. If we are rushed, brief, or **dismissive**, we may not make an emotional connection with the patient (**pathos**[2]). If we use **reasoning**, with data and words that are not understandable or logical (**logos**[3]) for the patient, then our connection with the patient is interrupted. The patient will be confused by the information we are providing and not appreciate our intentions.

Establishing an emotional connection with a patient always requires respect, time, and patience. I enter with a warm hello and open-ended questions and then try to

New Expressions	
rest on 基于；以……为基础	**ethos** /'iːθɑːs/ *n.* （某团体或社会的）道德思想，道德观
rhetorical /rɪ'tɔːrɪkl/ *adj.* 修辞的；修辞性的；带有修辞色彩的	**collapse** /kə'læps/ *v.* （突然）倒塌，坍塌
triangle /'traɪæŋgl/ *n.* 三角形；三角形物体	**dismissive** /dɪs'mɪsɪv/ *adj.* 轻蔑的；鄙视的
abrupt /ə'brʌpt/ *adj.* （言语、行为）粗鲁的，莽撞的，唐突的，生硬的	**reasoning** /'riːzənɪŋ/ *n.* 推想；推理；理性的观点；论证
off-putting /'ɔːf ˌpʊtɪŋ/ *adj.* 令人烦恼的；令人讨厌的	**logo** /'loʊɡoʊ/ *n.* （某公司或机构的）标识，标志，徽标
credible /'kredəbl/ *adj.* 可信的；可靠的	

---

① The text is adapted from the following source: Schraeder, T. L. 2019. *Physician Communication Connecting with Patients, Peers, and the Public*. New York: Oxford University Press.

assess the situation before we begin, **dipping** a toe in before we enter the pool of true interaction. I cannot assume anything about the patients' history, mood, or expectations until I spend time with them. I must be aware and cautious of first impressions and my own bias. Physician attitudes that can lead to poor communication include emotional burnout, **insecurity**, intolerance of diagnostic uncertainty, and negative bias toward specific health conditions. Inadequate training in psychosocial medicine and a limited knowledge of the patient's health condition can lead to difficult encounters. If we are anxious, depressed, exhausted, overworked, dealing with personal health issues or situational **stressors** or sleep **deprivation**, our patients will suffer; and if we have difficulty feeling and expressing empathy or are easily frustrated, we will not be good doctors.

While many physicians do not work in emergency situations requiring the level of communication to run a code, all of us work in unpredictable, stressful, emotional, and sometimes chaotic environments with individuals who we do not always fully know. We can learn from the underlying principles of the **Advanced Cardiovascular Life Support** (ACLS) training in our communication with patients and peers in any type of situation if we respect others, make sure our communications are clear and understood, make sure we fully understand what the other person is saying, and are willing to question, **converse**, and relate with **reverence**.

The following relationship building skills can be practiced by the doctors to have effective communication with their patients.

Show caring and warmth. There are so many nonphysical ways of showing warmth, from a smile to shared silence. Physical affection is not appropriate, of course, for a physician-patient relationship, and individuals react differently to different physical gestures from hugs to touching a shoulder or a hand. But we can certainly show kindness and caring by small and large gestures, from shaking hands to helping patients on and off the table. One person described how touched she was when a doctor who was caring for

New Expressions	
dip /dɪp/ *v.* 蘸；浸	**Advanced Cardiovascular Life Support** 高级心血管生命支持
insecurity /ˌɪnsɪˈkjʊrəti/ *n.* 心神不定；局促不安	
	converse /kənˈvɜːrs/ *v.* 交谈；谈话
stressor /ˈstresər/ *n.* 压力源	**reverence** /ˈrevərəns/ *n.* 尊敬；崇敬
deprivation /ˌdeprɪˈveɪʃn/ *n.* 剥夺；丧失；贫困	

her dying husband helped carry his shoes from one room to the next. Showing warmth toward a patient can come in a variety of nonphysical and professionally appropriate physical ways.

Be patient with each patient. If we are rushed or abrupt with patients, they are not going to feel cared for. If we cannot patiently listen, they will not feel we care. Just like with other relationships, we need to sit down and give them the time they need. Learning to make the most of the time you have and giving the patient your undivided attention for that time is key. Learning to listen and to accept your patients' unique qualities and never losing your curiosity about your patients or their lives are important. Learn how you can show respect to your patients, and you will learn more about them and how you can help them.

Listen carefully and thoughtfully. Be a good listener by leaning in, nodding, responding with "yes" or "uh-huh", and looking directly into your patients' eyes. Note not only the emotions of their words but also the cues of their body language.

Be thoughtful with small and large acts. Small acts can show you care. You can certainly show thoughtfulness by remembering important personal information about a patient's family. You can also pick up something they have dropped or ask them if they need a glass of water. Comment on the book they are reading or ask them what they are **knitting**. These interactions also give you a minute to put down your **stethoscope** and just relate human to human. Large acts of thoughtfulness mean going the extra mile in every aspect of their care. Take care of them as if they were a family member.

Show **gratitude**. Showing appreciation shows respect for the patients and their time. Thank patients for their questions. Thank them for sharing information with you. Thank them for coming to see you and being on time.

Be calm, gentle, and understanding. A calm, gentle, and understanding approach with most patients is much more beneficial than the opposite approach. Each patient is different. Each set of circumstances is different. We should remain gentle, open, humble, and understanding.

New Expressions	
knit /nɪt/ *v.* 编织；针织；机织	**gratitude** /'ɡrætɪtuːd/ *n.* 感激之情；感谢
stethoscope /'steθəskoʊp/ *n.* 听诊器	

Be open to their questions and ideas. Patients have their own concerns and ideas about their symptoms. They have their own ideas about the diagnosis and appropriate treatment. We need to elicit their thoughts, reasoning, and fears. We may know more about medicine, but they know more about their bodies, emotions, and lives than we do. Never assume you know everything about the patients or their symptoms, concerns, feelings, and lives.

Notes

1. **ethos**: 道德思想；道德观。它在文中代表可信性（credibility）、信任（trust）、尊敬（respect）和专业素质（professionalism）。
2. **pathos**: 感染力；令人产生悲悯共鸣的力量。它在文中代表情感（emotion）、共情（empathy）、人际关系（personal connection）和响应度（responsiveness）。
3. **logos**: 标识，标志，徽标。它在文中代表逻辑（logic）、推理（reasoning）、词汇（words）、数据（data）、结论（conclusions）和建议（recommendations）。

Post-reading Activities

I **Speaking Practice: Role Play**

Directions: *Please work in pairs. Imagine one of you is a doctor, and the other is a patient who has just been diagnosed with diabetes type 2. The patient is only about 36 years old and he/she found it difficult to accept the diagnosis. Please design a conversation between the doctor and the patient during which the doctor should deliver the news to the patient and respond to the patient's questions and needs in a proper manner. Be sure to use different strategies introduced in the text to maintain an effective doctor-patient communication. Please take turns to be the doctor and the patient.*

II Reflective Writing Practice: Mini-research Project

Directions: *Based on your reading and discussion, please follow the given steps and conduct a small-scale research project on the communication competence of medical students with your group members. Complete the following Research Report by filling out your major findings. Then reflect on your findings and write a short essay entitled "Communication Competence of Medical Students". The word limit is suggested to be 150–200 words.*

Research Report	
Research Objective	To investigate the communication competence of medical students
Research Method	Questionnaire
Research Procedures	1. Search and read literature on communication competence in general and the communication competence of medical students. 2. Design a questionnaire in reference to the prior literature and in response to your research objective. 3. Send at least 30 questionnaires to medical students in your university. 4. Collect the questionnaires. 5. Analyze the data.
Research Findings	Please summarize the findings based on your data analysis.

Unit 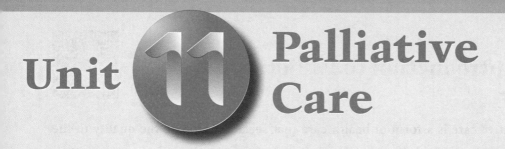 11 Palliative Care

> You matter because you are you, and you matter to the end of your life. We will do all we can not only to help you die peacefully, but also to live until you die.
>
> —Cicely Saunders

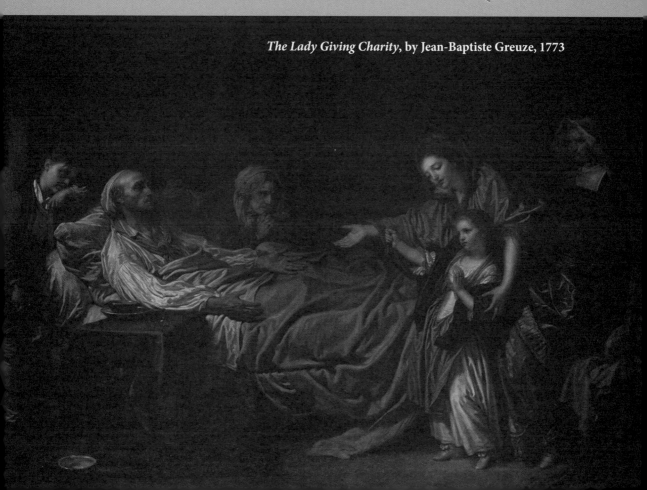

The Lady Giving Charity, by Jean-Baptiste Greuze, 1773

Part 1 Academic Horizon

An Introduction to Palliative Care[①][1]

Palliative care is a form of health care that seeks to improve the quality of life of patients with terminal disease through the prevention and relief of suffering. It is facilitated by the early identification of life-threatening disease and by the treatment of pain and disease-associated problems, including those that are physical, psychological, social, or spiritual in nature. As defined, palliative care begins at the point of diagnosis of terminal disease and can be delivered in a variety of health care settings. In general, it involves health and social care professionals working in hospitals, communities, hospices, and voluntary sectors.

Palliative care has been associated with many different terms, including terminal care, care of the dying, end-of-life care, and supportive care. However, these forms of care are not necessarily the same as palliative care. Likewise, palliative care is also sometimes described as **hospice care**[2]. While hospice care does imply palliative care, it is specific to care provided near the end of life. In contrast, palliative care covers the **duration** of a patient's illness and, hence, may be delivered over the course of years.

Principles of Palliative Care

Palliative care emphasizes three main principles:

- A team-based approach is fundamental in managing distressing symptoms, such as pain, **nausea**, **fatigue**, and depression. It is also a necessary component in meeting the physical and psychosocial needs of the patient

New Expressions	
palliative /ˈpæliətɪv/ *adj.*（治疗、药物）治标的，减轻痛苦的，缓解的	**nausea** /ˈnɔːsɪə/ *n.* 恶心；作呕；反胃
duration /duˈreɪʃn/ *n.* 持续时间；期间	**fatigue** /fəˈtiːɡ/ *n.* 疲劳；劳累

---

① The text is adapted from the following source: Kennedy, C. 2022. Palliative care. *Encyclopedia Britannica*. Retrieved November 13, 2022, from Encyclopedia Britannica website.

 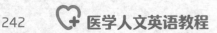 医学人文英语教程

and his/her family.

- Dying is a normal process. Symptom management is needed in order to help patients live life to the fullest until they die.

- The synthesis of physical care with psychological and spiritual care fulfills a vital role in the overall care of patients.

Types of Palliative Care

The concept of offering medical care for the dying within a setting organized for that purpose emerged in **Dublin**[3] in the late 19th century and was established in England early in the following century. The founding of the palliative care movement, however, is widely attributed to **Dame Cicely Saunders**[4], a British physician and humanitarian who pioneered the palliative care approach with the opening of **St. Christopher's Hospice**[5] in London in 1967. In the United Kingdom, it took two more decades for palliative care to be recognized as a medical specialty, and in the United States, it was not accepted as a medical discipline until 2006. Today, palliative care is recognized internationally, perhaps most importantly by the World Health Organization. Its acceptance as an area of medicine led to numerous advances in its delivery and to changes in its organization as a system of care. As a result, palliative care has been **subdivided** into general and specialist palliative care.

General palliative care is based on the three guiding principles of palliative care and is a core skill of nurses and doctors. The palliative care approach is a vital part of all clinical practice, regardless of patients' illness or its stage. It includes holistic consideration of patients and the needs of the patients' family, in addition to addressing medical and physical concerns. General palliative care is delivered on the basis of need, not diagnosis and is delivered in hospitals, in patients' homes, or in specialized care facilities, such as **nursing homes**.

Specialists in palliative care deliver care for patients with complex needs. Specialist palliative care teams are **multidisciplinary**, being composed of nurses, doctors, **allied**

New Expressions	
synthesis /'sɪnθəsɪs/ *n.* 综合；结合；综合体	**multidisciplinary** /ˌmʌltɪ'dɪsəpləneri/ *adj.*（涉及）多门学科的
subdivide /ˌsʌbdɪ'vaɪd/ *v.*（被）再分割，再分	**allied** /'ælaɪd/ *adj.*（两个或以上事物）类似的，共存的，有关联的
nursing home 养老院	

health and social care professionals, religious leaders, and individuals from the voluntary sector. Specialists may be based in a hospice or may be part of a specialist team at a hospital. They work either directly with patients and families or with other health care professionals to complement the general care that patients receive. Their work may be carried out in hospitals, community care facilities, or patients' homes.

Hospice Care

Hospice care, which is concerned with the delivery of medical, psychological, and spiritual support near the end of a patient's life, developed largely from the work of **charitable** organizations. Today hospice facilities provide a variety of services, including specialist and community palliative care. In addition, hospice care may be delivered in any of several different settings, including at hospice inpatient units, in hospitals or nursing homes with hospice beds, at a patient's home, or at a hospice **day care**.

Hospice inpatient units were initially established to deal with the needs of patients suffering from terminal cancer. Hospice services increasingly have been sought from patients with other terminal illnesses, such as **amyotrophic lateral sclerosis**[6] (ALS; motor neuron disease). Children's hospices have been developed for the needs of children requiring palliative care for conditions, such as degenerative or malignant disease.

Patients are admitted to inpatient hospice care for a variety of reasons, including assessment, **rehabilitation**, pain and symptom management, and short **respite stays**[7] or terminal care. Families are encouraged to be involved in care where appropriate, and visiting tends to be open. Staff normally have access to specialized training and education in palliative care.

Developments in Palliative Care

Palliative care is a global concern, and a steady rise in the number of people who are living longer with degenerative disease suggests that demand for palliative care services will increase in the 21st century. In some places, palliative care standards are incorporated into a larger system of care. For example, the **Gold Standards Framework**[8] offers guidance to primary health care teams and has identified tasks that help improve

New Expressions	
charitable /'tʃærətəbl/ *adj.* 慈善团体的；慈善事业的	**rehabilitation** /ˌriːəˌbɪlɪ'teɪʃn/ *n.* 康复
day care 日间护理	**respite** /'respɪt/ *n.* 暂停；暂缓

end-of-life care in the community. Thus, the framework is intended to be used throughout a patient's illness rather than only in the last days of life. Its principles reflect those of the WHO and include symptom control, effective communication, coordination and continuity in services, support and care of the dying and their families, and continued learning for staff.

Notes

1. **Palliative Care:** 缓和医疗。根据《英国医学杂志》(*BMJ*)中文版编委会 2017 年组织的关于 palliative care 和 hospice care 中文翻译的圆桌讨论会，palliative care 的中文翻译用"缓和医疗"替代"姑息治疗"，hospice care 的中文翻译用"安宁疗护"替代"临终关怀"，更容易被公众接受。安宁疗护是缓和医疗最后的重要阶段，而非全部。世界卫生组织将缓和医疗 / 姑息治疗定义为"提高那些面临危及生命的疾病相关问题的（成人和儿童）患者及其家人的生活质量的一种办法。这种治疗通过早期识别、正确评估和处理疼痛及其他身体、社会心理或精神问题，预防并减轻痛苦"。Palliative care is, as defined by the World Health Organization, "an approach that improves the quality of life of patients (adults and children) and their families who are facing problems associated with life-threatening illness. It prevents and relieves suffering through the early identification, correct assessment, and treatment of pain and other problems, whether physical, psychosocial, or spiritual."

2. **hospice care:** 安宁疗护。中华人民共和国国家卫生健康委员会于 2017 年 1 月发布的《安宁疗护实践指南（试行）》将安宁疗护实践定义为"以临终患者和家属为中心，以多学科协作模式进行，主要内容包括疼痛及其他症状控制，舒适照护，心理、精神及社会支持等"。

3. **Dublin:** 都柏林。都柏林是爱尔兰共和国首都，临爱尔兰海，位于利菲河口。Dublin is the capital city of the Republic of Ireland, situated on the Irish Sea at the mouth of the River Liffey.

4. **Dame Cicely Saunders:** 西西里·桑德斯女爵士，1918—2005。Cicely Saunders founded the first modern hospice and, more than anybody else, was responsible for establishing the discipline and the culture of palliative care. She introduced effective pain management and insisted that dying people needed dignity, compassion, and respect, as well as rigorous scientific methodology in the testing of treatments.

5. St. Christopher's Hospice: 圣·克里斯托弗安宁院。St. Christopher's Hospice was founded by Dame Cicely Saunders in 1967 and is widely recognized as the first modern hospice.

6. amyotrophic lateral sclerosis: 肌萎缩侧索硬化症。Amyotrophic lateral sclerosis (ALS) is progressive degeneration of the motor neurons of the central nervous system, leading to wasting of the muscles and paralysis.

7. respite stays: 短期停留，暂时托管。这是为老人、精神病患者等提供的短期照料，以使长期照顾者获得短暂休息，也被称为 respite care。Respite stay is the temporary care arranged for old, mentally ill, etc. people so that the people who usually care for them can have a rest.

8. Gold Standards Framework: 金标准框架。20 世纪初，凯利·托马斯（Keri Thomas）教授创立了"金标准框架"，旨在提升社区安宁疗护服务的质量。The Gold Standards Framework (GSF) is an evidence-based systematic approach to formalizing best practice through improving the organization and coordination of care for all people with any condition in any setting in the final year or so of life.

Post-reading Activities

I Speaking Practice: Group Discussion

Directions: *Please discuss the following questions in small groups. After your discussion, please share your opinions with the whole class.*

1. What ideas would come to your mind when you hear the two terms "palliative care" and "hospice care"?

2. According to the text, what are the differences between palliative care and hospice care?

3. What is general palliative care? What is specialist palliative care?

II Speaking Practice: Oral Presentation

Directions: *Please search for information on the development of palliative care provided in the mainland, Hong Kong, Macao, and Taiwan of China. And then give an oral presentation to introduce your findings to the whole class.*

Part 2 Thematic Reading

A Personal Therapeutic Journey①

I began training as a ward nurse in 1941 at St. Thomas's Hospital. We had a limited **pharmacopoeia**, which gradually included **sulphonamides** but no other antibiotics, and few of the other drugs that we now take for granted. **Invalided** out with back trouble, I returned to Oxford in 1944, had a **laminectomy**, and became a medical social worker back at St. Thomas's.

Brompton Cocktails[1]

In March 1948, I began working as a volunteer nurse once or twice a week in one of the early homes for "terminal care". St. Luke's Hospital had 48 beds for patients with **advanced** cancer. Here I met the regular administration of a modified "Brompton cocktail". From 1951 to 1957, I was a medical student, yet again at St. Thomas's. During that time there was a revolution in the drugs available for control of symptoms. The first **phenothiazines**, the antidepressants, the **benzodiazepines**, the **synthetic steroids**, and the **nonsteroidal anti-inflammatory drugs**[2] had all come into use by the time I arrived at St. Joseph's Hospice in October 1958. St. Joseph's Irish Sisters of Charity had welcomed the local chest physician with the new **antituberculosis** drugs in the early 1950s and

New Expressions	
pharmacopoeia /ˌfɑːrməkəˈpiːə/ *n.* 药典；备用药品	氮卓类药物（二类精神药物）
sulphonamide /sʌlˈfɒnəmaɪd/ *n.* 磺胺类药物	**synthetic** /sɪnˈθetɪk/ *adj.* 人造的；（人工）合成的
invalid /ˈɪnvəliːd/ *v.* （因伤病）令⋯⋯退役	**steroid** /ˈstɪrɔɪd/ *n.* 甾族化合物；类固醇
laminectomy /læmɪˈnektəmi/ *n.* 椎板切除术	**nonsteroidal** /ˌnɑːnstɪˈrɔɪdl/ *adj.* 非甾类化合物的；非类固醇的
advanced /ədˈvænst/ *adj.* （发展）晚期的，后期的	**anti-inflammatory** /ˌænti ɪnˈflæmətɔri/ *adj.* 消炎的；抗炎的
phenothiazine /ˌfiːnoʊˈθaɪəˌzin/ *n.* 吩噻嗪（用作杀虫剂或药物制造）	**antituberculosis** /ˌæntituːˌbɜːrkjəˈloʊsɪs/ *adj.* （药物等）抗结核的
benzodiazepine /ˌbenzoʊdaɪˈæzəˌpin/ *n.* 苯二	

---

① The text is adapted from the following source: Saunders, C. 1996. A personal therapeutic journey. *British Medical Journal*, 313(7072): 1599–1601.

were ready for further innovations. Oral morphine together with alcohol and **cocaine** was introduced with **cyclizine** as the main **antiemetic**. The therapeutic advances and having the time to sit and listen to a patient's story, transformed the wards.

Greater Confidence

We had by that time begun to use **diamorphine**. There were no controlled trials of this drug to be found, only some clinical reports that it had few side effects. We used it for 42 of our first 500 patients, in women with severe nausea and in a few patients with **intolerable** feelings of **suffocation**. By that time, we believed that this was the drug of choice, but I realized two things. Firstly, we were getting better and more confident in all that we were doing. Secondly, our own enthusiasms must be tested.

During the seven years at St. Joseph's between 1958 and 1965, we increased our pharmacopoeia, our patients' activities, their **discharges**, and referrals back for **radiotherapy**. I wrote and lectured widely and produced a handout of the drugs in common use at St. Joseph's and at St. Christopher's Hospice, which opened in 1967.

It soon became clear that each death was as individual as the life that preceded it and that the whole experience of that life was reflected in a patient's dying. This led to the concept of "total pain", which was presented as a complex of physical, emotional, social, and spiritual elements. The whole experience for a patient includes anxiety, depression, and fear; concern for the family who will become **bereaved**; and often a need to find some meaning in the situation, some deeper reality in which to trust. This became the major emphasis of much lecturing and writing on subjects, such as the nature and management of terminal pain and the family as the unit of care.

Importance of Active Total Care

It was recognized that support was needed both before and after a patient's death, particularly in home care, when the family are the central carers. The World Health

---

New Expressions

cocaine /kou'keɪn/ *n.* 可卡因；古柯碱

cyclizine /'saɪkləˌzɪn/ *n.* 赛克利嗪；苯甲嗪（止吐剂，治晕动病）

antiemetic /ˌæntiiˈmetɪk/ *n.* 止吐剂

diamorphine /ˌdaɪəˈmɔːrfiːn/ *n.* 二乙酰吗啡，海洛因（用以镇痛）

intolerable /ɪnˈtɑːlərəbl/ *adj.* 无法忍受的；不能容忍的；完全不可接受的

suffocation /ˌsʌfəˈkeɪʃn/ *n.* 窒息

discharge /dɪsˈtʃɑːrdʒ/ *n.* 出院

radiotherapy /ˌreɪdiouˈθerəpi/ *n.* 放射疗法

bereaved /bɪˈriːvd/ *adj.* 丧失亲友的

Organization has published the following definition, "Palliative care is the active total care of patients whose disease is not responsive to **curative** treatment. Control of pain, of other symptoms and of psychological, social and spiritual problems is paramount. The goal of palliative care is achievement of the best possible quality of life for patients and their families."

The basic and clinical researchers, together with many clinicians—doctors, nurses, and many in **auxiliary** services—have enlarged our detailed knowledge of physical pain since that was written. The emphasis on regular giving has been accepted widely and also features as an essential element in relieving the pain of cancer. Over 33 years later, these basic principles have not changed, although symptomatic treatment is far more complex and specialists in palliative care have to **keep abreast of** developments in all relevant disciplines.

Many therapeutic discoveries of recent years have been relevant to palliative care. **Neuropathic** pain is better managed but still needs further work. Looking ahead, I sometimes wonder that if we are not careful, we may see a post-antibiotic era. Whatever happens, it will still matter that we go on listening and that we continue our questioning. Above all, my experience emphasizes that the practice of medicine includes more than specific treatments.

We Were the Hosts

The advances in **pharmacology** and the new technologies are not the whole story. At our preliminary training school, we were taught that we were host to our patients and their visiting families. Life has changed greatly in over 55 years, but people's needs, though expressed differently, remain beyond the strictly physical. Palliative care physicians are not to be merely "**symptomatologists**", as Kearney has expressed it.

Now that palliative care is spreading worldwide, it has still, as in the WHO definition, kept a concern for the spiritual needs of its patients and their families. The

New Expressions	
curative /'kjʊrətɪv/ *adj.* 能治病的；有疗效的	**pharmacology** /ˌfɑːrmə'kɑːlədʒi/ *n.* 药物学；药理学
auxiliary /ɔːg'zɪliəri/ *adj.* 辅助的	
keep abreast of 了解……的最新情况	**symptomatologist** /ˌsɪmptəmə'tɑlədʒɪst/ *n.* 症候学家；症状学家
neuropathic /ˌnjʊrə'pæθɪk/ *adj.* 神经病的；神经性的	

whole approach has been based on the understanding that a person is an **indivisible** entity, a physical and a spiritual being. "The only proper response to a person is respect; a way of seeing and listening to each one in the whole context of their culture and relationships, thereby giving each his/her **intrinsic** value." The search for meaning, for something in which to trust, may be expressed in many ways, direct and indirect, in **metaphor** or silence, in gesture or symbol, or, perhaps most of all, in art and the unexpected potential for creativity at the end of life. Those who work in palliative care may have to realize that they, too, are being challenged to face this dimension for themselves. If we can come not only in our professional capacity but in our common, vulnerable humanity, there may be no need of words on our part, only of concerned listening. For those who do not wish to share their deepest needs, the way care is given can reach the most hidden places. Feelings of fear and guilt may seem **inconsolable**, but many of us have sensed that an inner journey has taken place and that a person nearing the end of life has found peace. Important relationships may be developed or **reconciled** at this time and a new sense of **self-worth** develops.

My personal therapeutic journey has witnessed an extraordinary growth in drug treatments for pain and other symptoms. The challenge of educating others on their use remains. However, there has always been a human as well as a professional basis that is fundamental to the work that we do. Everyone meeting these patients and their families is challenged to have some awareness of this dimension. Professionals' own search for meaning can create a climate, as we tried often helplessly to do all those years ago, in which patients and families can reach out in trust towards what they see as true and find courage and acceptance of what is happening to them.

New Expressions

indivisible /ˌɪndɪ'vɪzəbl/ *adj.* 分不开的；不可分割的

inconsolable /ˌɪnkən'soʊləbl/ *adj.* 悲痛欲绝的；无法慰藉的

intrinsic /ɪn'trɪnsɪk/ *adj.* 固有的；内在的；本身的

reconcile /'rekənsaɪl/ *v.* 使和解；使和好如初

self-worth /ˌself 'wɜːrθ/ *n.* 自我价值感

metaphor /'metəfɔːr/ *n.* 暗喻；隐喻

Notes

1. **Brompton Cocktails:** 布朗普顿混合麻醉剂。布朗普顿混合麻醉剂用以减轻癌症末期的疼痛，以首次使用本药剂的伦敦皇家布朗普顿胸科医院而命名。The Brompton cocktail is an oral analgesic mixture of morphine, heroin, cocaine, chloroform, ethyl alcohol, and flavored syrup, first used in the 1920s at the Royal Brompton Chest Hospital in London for patients with tuberculosis. It was subsequently repurposed and genericized, and refers to any alcoholic solution containing an opioid (heroin or morphine) and either cocaine or a phenothiazine to improve the quality of life in terminally ill cancer patients.

2. **nonsteroidal anti-inflammatory drugs:** 非甾体抗炎药。非甾体抗炎药是一类抗炎作用不同于皮质激素类而具有抗炎、解热和镇痛作用的药物，在临床上广泛用于骨关节炎、类风湿性关节炎和多种免疫功能紊乱的炎症性疾病及各种疼痛（如牙痛、头痛、痛经及肌肉痛）症状的缓解，是全世界范围内使用最广泛的一类药物。阿司匹林是非甾体抗炎药的典型代表。Nonsteroidal anti-inflammatory drugs (NSAIDs) refer to a group of medicines that relieve pain and fever, and reduce inflammation.

Post-reading Activities

I Language Building-up

Task 1 Extensive Vocabulary Enlargement

Directions: *The following words are taken from the text. Please follow the three-step learning in this part and build up your own Extensive Vocabulary Chart.*

Step 1. Read through the words and underline them in the text. Circle the ones that are particularly new to you. Look up the words in the dictionary and put the equivalent Chinese translation in the chart on the next page.

Step 2. While you go back to the text, please feel free to put any other words into the blanks provided in the extra lines in the chart.

Extensive Vocabulary Chart				
pharmacopoeia	sulphonamide	invalid	laminectomy	phenothiazine
benzodiazepine	steroid	anti-inflammatory	antituberculosis	cocaine
cyclizine	antiemetic	diamorphine	suffocation	radiotherapy
curative	neuropathic	pharmacology	symptomatologist	self-worth

Step 3. Please group the above words based on their parts of speech and meanings.

Nouns	
Verbs	
Adjectives	
Adverbs and Prepositions	
Medical Terminology	
Terminology in Other Fields	

Directions: *The following 10 words are chosen from the text. They will form the intensive vocabulary in this unit. For intensive vocabulary, you are supposed to be able to explain them in English and use them in sentence and discourse constructions.*

Step 1.　Please read through the words and be familiar with their Chinese and English definitions. Recall where and how they are used in the text.

No.	Word	Translation	Definition	Status
			Intensive Vocabulary Chart	
1	synthetic	人造的;（人工）合成的	*adj.* artificial; made by combining chemical substances rather than being produced naturally by plants or animals	☆☆☆☆☆
2	intolerable	无法忍受的；不能容忍的；完全不可接受的	*adj.* so bad or difficult that you cannot tolerate it; completely unacceptable	☆☆☆☆☆
3	discharge	出院	*n.* the act of allowing sb. to leave the hospital because he/she is well enough to leave	☆☆☆☆☆
4	bereaved	丧失亲友的	*adj.* having lost a relative or close friend who has recently died	☆☆☆☆☆
5	auxiliary	辅助的	*adj.* giving help or support to the main group of workers	☆☆☆☆☆
6	indivisible	分不开的；不可分割的	*adj.* that cannot be divided into separate parts	☆☆☆☆☆
7	intrinsic	固有的；内在的；本身的	*adj.* belonging to or part of the real nature of sth./sb.	☆☆☆☆☆
8	metaphor	暗喻；隐喻	*n.* a word or phrase used to describe sb./sth. else, in a way that is different from its normal use, in order to show that the two things have the same qualities and to make the description more powerful	☆☆☆☆☆
9	inconsolable	悲痛欲绝的；无法慰藉的	*adj.* very sad and unable to accept help or comfort	☆☆☆☆☆
10	reconcile	使和解；使好如初	*v.* to make people become friends again after an argument or a disagreement	☆☆☆☆☆

Step 2.　Please tick the status for each word based on your own situation. If one word is very new or difficult for you, please tick five stars. Likewise, if one word is

comparatively easy for you and you don't have to spend too much time on reading and learning it, then tick one star. The number of stars represents the difficulty of commanding a word in your eyes.

Step 3. Please complete the following 10 sentences by choosing appropriate words from the Intensive Vocabulary Chart. Please change the forms of the words where necessary.

1. Nurses visit the mother and baby for two weeks after their _____ from the hospital.

2. The pair were _____ after Jackson made a public apology.

3. The job placed almost _____ pressure on her.

4. Far from being separate, the mind and body form a(n) _____ whole.

5. Boots made from _____ materials can usually be washed in a machine.

6. Flexibility is _____ to creative management.

7. Mr. Dinkins visited the _____ family to offer comfort.

8. They were _____ when their only child died.

9. In poetry the rose is often a(n) _____ for love.

10. The government's first concern was to augment the army and _____ forces.

Task 3   Expressions and Sentences

Directions: *The following sentences are taken from the text. In each sentence, there is one phrase being underlined. Please refer to the dictionary and write down the explanation of the phrase in the line entitled "Meaning Exploration". After that, please make a sentence with it. Write the sentence in the line entitled "Sentence Making".*

Sentence 1

Original Sentence	We had a limited pharmacopoeia, which gradually included sulphonamides but no other antibiotics, and few of the other drugs that we now take for granted.
Meaning Exploration	*take (sth.) for granted*:
Sentence Making	

Sentence 2

Original Sentence	I wrote and lectured widely and produced a handout of the drugs <u>in common use</u> at St. Joseph's and at St. Christopher's Hospice, which opened in 1967.
Meaning Exploration	*in common use:*
Sentence Making	

Sentence 3

Original Sentence	Over 33 years later, these basic principles have not changed, although symptomatic treatment is far more complex and specialists in palliative care have to <u>keep abreast of</u> developments in all relevant disciplines.
Meaning Exploration	*keep abreast of:*
Sentence Making	

Sentence 4

Original Sentence	Important relationships may be developed or reconciled at this time and <u>a</u> new <u>sense of</u> self-worth develops.
Meaning Exploration	*a sense of:*
Sentence Making	

Sentence 5

Original Sentence	However, there has always been a human <u>as well as</u> a professional basis that is fundamental to the work that we do.
Meaning Exploration	*as well as:*
Sentence Making	

II Critical Reading and Thinking

Task 1   Overview and Comprehension

Directions: *The main body of the text could be divided into four small sections in line with the four given subtitles. Please write down the main information provided in each part based on your reading.*

Reading Notes	
Brompton Cocktails	
Greater Confidence	
Importance of Active Total Care	
We Were the Hosts	

Task 2   Reflection and Discussion

Directions: *After reading, please reflect on the theme of the text. Work in groups and share your opinions on the following questions with other group members.*

1. Why did the author say that the therapeutic advances and having the time to sit and listen to a patient's story transformed the wards?

2. What is total pain according to the author Cicely Saunders?

3. What might be the reasons that "support was needed both before and after a patient's death"? How can you offer bereavement support for grieving families?

4. In the last paragraph, Cicely Saunders stated that "there has always been a human as well as a professional basis that is fundamental to the work that we do". What do you think the human and professional basis of palliative care is?

Part 3 Extended Reading

The Challenge of Knowing[①]

I had just finished rounding in the hospital when the phone rang.

"Something is wrong. The doctor is here. Talk to him," she said to me from my father's bedside. The **cardiologist** got on the phone, and he must have told me about the **myocardial infarction**[1] or the **hypotension**, but all I heard was "emergency **heart catheterization**[2]".

The last time I saw him was just three hours ago. I had made a special trip to the hospital across town before work, so I could be there when the doctors were on their ward rounds. He and I joked about how unhealthful the hospital breakfast seemed. He called me his little girl and told me that I didn't need to sit there with him. He told me he was fine. He told me he loved me.

I set the phone down and packed my bag, leaving the hospital without even saying goodbye to my colleagues. The 10-minute drive took years. The subsequent hours in the tiny waiting room took decades. I had flashbacks to residency when I coded a patient outside the **cardiac** catheter laboratory, but this time the patient had my father's face. A **revolving** door of physicians **floated** unfamiliar words at us, including things that didn't exist widely when I was in residency, such as "**intubation**" and "ECMO (**extracorporeal membrane oxygenation**)[3]". I took off my daughter hat and hid behind my physician

New Expressions	
cardiologist /ˌkɑːrdiˈɑːlədʒɪst/ *n.* 心脏病医生；心脏病学家	**revolving** /rɪˈvɔːlvɪŋ/ *adj.* 旋转的
myocardial /ˌmaɪoʊˈkɑrdiəl/ *adj.* 心肌的	**float** /floʊt/ *v.* 提出，提请考虑（想法或计划）
infarction /ɪnˈfɑːrkʃn/ *n.* 梗死	**intubation** /ˌɪntjəˈbeɪʃn/ *n.* 插管
hypotension /ˌhaɪpəˈtenʃn/ *n.* 低血压	**extracorporeal** /ˌekstrəkɔːrˈpɔːriəl/ *adj.*（位于或发生在）体外的
catheterization /ˌkæθɪtəraɪˈzeɪʃn/ *n.* 导管插入术	**oxygenation** /ˌɑːksɪdʒəˈneɪʃn/ *n.* 充氧；氧合作用
cardiac /ˈkɑːrdiæk/ *adj.* 心脏的；心脏病的	

---

① The text is adapted from the following source: Kalender-Rich, J. 2021. The challenge of knowing. *JAMA*, *325*(21): 2155–2156.

armor, researching the newer technology, calling my hospital to arrange a transfer.

When we got to my hospital, I felt like I was back home. I had no idea how comforting it would be to recognize the wallpaper and know where the bathroom was without asking. The next few days were a blur of procedures and teams of specialists, high-tech machines and numbers, family and friends. I was a daughter and a doctor—a **geriatrician** and a palliative care physician, an **internist**. I looked at the numbers. I looked at the faces of the bedside team. I hoped and I prayed and I paced. And deep in my soul I knew. But my family didn't.

Over the next ten days, I interpreted the medical **jargon** for family and friends. I stayed in the hospital waiting room day after day and night after night. I had flashbacks of calling families just like mine right after they went home to tell them their loved one was worse. I became a **fixture** in his **intensive care unit (ICU)**[4] room and asked hundreds of questions. I left my pager number and cell number, but I never left the building. Because I knew.

I asked the ICU attending his opinion on the case and made him promise to call me with changes. I **hovered** every morning when the team rounded in the hopes of **overhearing** anything that my physician mind could lean on. I **hounded** the fellow who was once my medical student, asking **pointed** questions about recovery potential. Because I knew.

Through it all, the medical team did their job. They used every tool in their **kits** to try to save him. They marched along looking for answers. And then they set a deadline, a day they planned to try to **wean** the ECMO **circuit**. They strategically avoided my questions about the **prognosis**. I looked at my father, and I thought back to conversations

New Expressions	
armor /'ɑːrmər/ *n.* 盔甲	hound /haʊnd/ *v.* 追踪；追逐；纠缠
geriatrician /ˌdʒeriə'trɪʃn/ *n.* 老年病科医师；老年病学专家	pointed /'pɔɪntɪd/ *adj.* 尖锐的；尖刻的
	kit /kɪt/ *n.* 成套工具；成套设备
internist /ɪn'tɜːrnɪst/ *n.* 内科医生	wean /wiːn/ *v.* 使逐渐戒除某些习惯（或使用某些东西）
jargon /'dʒɑːrɡən/ *n.* 行话；行业术语	
fixture /'fɪkstʃər/ *n.* 固定成员；固定设施	circuit /'sɜːrkɪt/ *n.* 电路；线路
hover /'hʌvər/ *v.* 踌躇，彷徨（尤指在某人身边）	prognosis /prɑːɡ'noʊsɪs/ *n.* （对病情的）预断，预后
overhear /ˌoʊvər'hɪr/ *v.* 偶然听到；无意中听到	

we had over the years, in which he had **disdainfully** talked about being dependent on others even for a short time. I thought about my own patients and their **protracted** recovery times in long-term acute care hospitals, and I knew.

The night before the planned weaning trial, I recalled what I had told so many suffering families. I leaned over him, told him that I loved him, and told him that he was in charge. I told him that we would be okay and would support whatever decision he made. I told him that it was up to him to give us some answers.

And then I waited.

Physicians often enter medicine to improve people's lives and help them live better, but somewhere along the way, we get lost in organ systems and disease. We drown in frequent laboratory reports and **fluctuating** vital signs. And we lose the bigger picture. There are times when we look at a patient and, in the back of our minds, think "Poor guy. There is no way he can fully recover from this." But we don't tell the patient or family because we are the fixers. We are the healers who came to this noble profession to cure the sick and fix the disease. We cannot fail. This is the tragedy. Only when we take a step back and look at the entire person can we really see them. Only then are we treating patients instead of body parts.

Every month I take fourth-year medical students through a **high-fidelity mannequin simulation** during which they practice telling a **standardized patient**[5] actor that their loved one is dying. I give them examples of phrases to use when sharing difficult information and body language to convey empathy. I ask them to **put themselves in the family's shoes** and question when and how they would want to be told their loved one may not survive. Suddenly, I was the family waiting to be told.

I often wonder when the medical team suspected he would probably die; I assume it was long before they started the conversation. I'm sure this was well-intentioned.

New Expressions	
disdainfully /dɪs'deɪnfəli/ *adv.* 轻视地；鄙视地；倨傲地	**high-fidelity** /ˌhaɪ fɪ'deləti/ *adj.* 高保真度的
	mannequin /'mænɪkɪn/ *n.* 人体模型
protracted /prə'træktɪd/ *adj.* 延长的；拖延的；持久的	**simulation** /ˌsɪmju'leɪʃn/ *n.* 模拟；仿真
fluctuate /'flʌktʃueɪt/ *v.* （大小、数量、质量等）波动；（在……之间）起伏不定	**put oneself in one's shoes** 设身处地为他人着想；换位思考

Sometimes, though, the family knows before the doctors. Sometimes they are just waiting for the doctors to **confirm** their fears. Sometimes they know.

As I both feared and somehow expected, my father took my **whispered** statements seriously and left no room for us to wonder about next steps. His rapid **decline** the next morning was followed by hours of transfusions, medications, and finally, "the talk". The doctors were now answering the questions they previously **sidestepped**. The family gathered to his bedside and only after everyone had arrived to provide each other comfort did my father find his own peace.

Days later we began the process of updating bank accounts. We found the notes from one week before his first procedure when he, for the first time ever, had shared his passwords with my mother. Because he also knew.

New Expressions

confirm /kən'fɜːrm/ v. (尤指提供证据来) 证实，证明，确认

whisper /'wɪspər/ v. 耳语；低语；小声说

decline /dɪ'klaɪn/ n. (数量、价值、质量等的) 减少，下降，衰落，衰退

sidestep /'saɪdstep/ v. 回避，规避 (问题等)

Notes

1. **myocardial infarction:** 心肌梗死。心肌梗死是由心脏供血的中断而引起的心肌层部位的坏死，分急性期、亚急性期和慢性期三期。临床症状主要出现在急性期，表现多是持续性剧烈的胸骨后疼痛，服用硝酸甘油不能缓解，严重者会出现休克、心律失常、心力衰竭的现象。Myocardial infarction refers to necrosis of a region of the myocardium caused by an interruption in the supply of blood to the heart.

2. **heart catheterization:** 心脏导管检查。心脏导管检查是将不能被 X 线透过的心脏导管在透视下送入心脏各腔和大血管，进行有关血液动力学及血气分析等检查，借以诊断心脏病。Heart catheterization, also known as cardiac catheterization, is a procedure in which a thin, flexible tube (catheter) is guided through a blood vessel to the heart to diagnose or treat certain heart conditions, such as clogged arteries or irregular heartbeats. Heart catheterization gives doctors important information about the heart muscle, heart valves, and blood vessels in the heart.

3. **ECMO (extracorporeal membrane oxygenation):** 体外膜肺氧合。体外膜肺氧合是一种医疗急救设备，用以暂时协助大部分医疗方法皆无效的重度心肺衰竭患者

进行体外的呼吸与循环。In intensive care medicine, extracorporeal membrane oxygenation is an extracorporeal technique of providing both cardiac and respiratory support to persons whose heart and lungs are unable to provide an adequate amount of gas exchange to sustain life.

4. **intensive care unit (ICU):** 重症监护病房。重症监护病房是指把需要特别治疗和护理的急、重症病人集中收容的一个专设的病区或病室，在其中使用专门诊疗技术和仪器设备对病人实施加强诊疗、护理和监护。Intensive care unit is a specialized section of a hospital containing the equipment, medical and nursing staff, and monitoring devices necessary to provide intensive care.

5. **standardized patient:** 标准化病人。标准化病人是现代医学教育测量专用语，是指那些经过标准化、系统化训练后，能准确表现病人的实际临床问题的正常人或病人。标准化病人是医学教育测量中的特殊手段，已广泛应用于医学教育各领域，从医学生的交流技能到临床医疗质量的评估。它应用的范围包括问诊、身体检查、模仿病人的某些症状和阳性体征。In health care, a standardized patient (SP), also known as a simulated patient, is an individual trained to act as a real patient in order to simulate a set of symptoms or problems. Standardized patients have been successfully utilized for education, evaluation of health care professionals, and basic, applied and translational medical research.

Post-reading Activities

I **Speaking Practice: Role Play**

Directions: *Please work in pairs. Imagine one of you is a doctor, and the other is a close family member of a terminal patient. Please design a conversation between the doctor and the family member during which the doctor tries to tell the family member of the terminal patient that his/her loved one is dying. Be sure to use effective phrases and proper body language to break bad news and convey empathy. Please take turns to be the doctor and the close family member.*

Phrases to break bad news:

1. _____

2. _____

3. _____

Body language to convey empathy:

1. _____

2. _____

3. _____

▌ Reflective Writing Practice: Mini-research Project

Directions: *Based on your reading and discussion, please follow the given steps and conduct a small-scale research project on people's knowledge of and attitude towards palliative care with your group members. Complete the following Research Report by filling out your major findings. Then reflect on your findings and write a short essay entitled "Knowledge of and Attitude Towards Palliative Care". The word limit is suggested to be 150–200 words.*

Research Report	
Research Objective	To investigate people's knowledge of and attitude towards palliative care
Research Method	Interview
Research Procedures	1. Search and read literature on palliative care both at home and abroad. 2. Design an interview outline which includes several questions about people's knowledge of and attitude towards palliative care. 3. Interview at least five people based on your interview outline. Record the interview after gaining consent from the interviewees. 4. Analyze the interview data.
Research Findings	Please summarize the findings based on your data analysis.

Unit 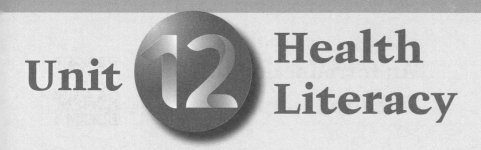 Health Literacy

> To deliver high-quality, safe, and high-value care, health care systems must provide information that people can easily find, understand, and use. Health literacy tools can help systems deliver person-centered care.
>
> —Gopal Khanna

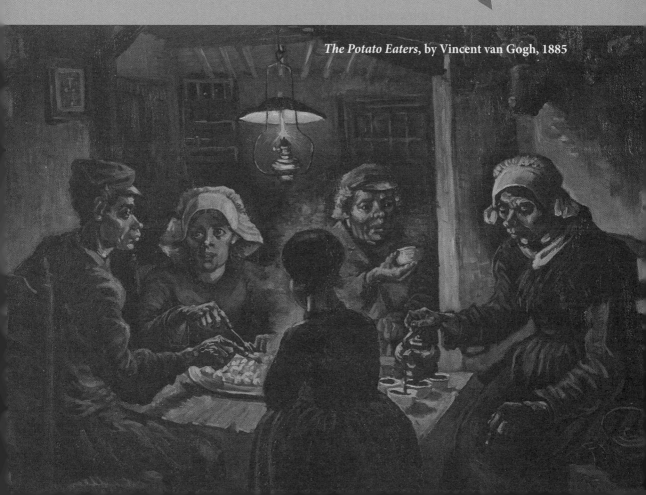

The Potato Eaters, by Vincent van Gogh, 1885

Part 1 Academic Horizon

An Introduction to Health Literacy①

What Is Health Literacy?

According to **the U.S. Department of Health and Human Services (HHS)**[1] **Healthy People 2030**[2] initiative, health literacy involves the information and services that people need to make **well-informed** health decisions. There are many aspects of health literacy:

- Personal health literacy is the degree to which individuals have the ability to find, understand, and use information and services to inform health-related decisions and actions for themselves and others. Examples of personal health literacy include understanding prescription drug instructions, understanding doctors' directions and **consent forms**, and the ability to navigate the complex health care system.

- Organizational health literacy is the degree to which organizations equitably enable individuals to find, understand, and use information and services to inform health-related decisions and actions for themselves and others. Examples of organizational health literacy include **simplifying** the process to schedule appointments, using **the Teach-Back method**[3] to ensure patient comprehension, and providing communications in the appropriate language, reading level, and format.

- Digital health literacy, as defined by the World Health Organization, is the

New Expressions	
well-informed /wel ɪn'fɔːrmd/ *adj.* 见多识广的；消息灵通的；知识渊博的	**consent form** 知情同意书
	simplify /'sɪmplɪfaɪ/ *v.* 使简化；使简易

---

① The text is adapted from the following source: National Library of Medicine. n.d. An introduction to health literacy. *National Library of Medicine*. Retrieved December 19, 2022, from National Library of Medicine website.

 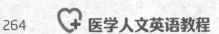

ability to seek, find, understand, and appraise health information from electronic sources and apply the knowledge gained to addressing or solving a health problem. Examples of digital health literacy include accessing your electronic health record, communicating electronically with your health care team, ability to **discern** reliable online health information, and using health and **wellness** apps.

- **Numeracy**, also known as quantitative literacy, refers to a set of mathematical and advanced problem-solving skills that are necessary to succeed in a society increasingly driven by data, as defined by **the National Association of Secondary School Principals**[4]. Examples of numeracy include understanding nutrition information, interpreting **blood sugar** readings, taking a correct **dosage** of medication (for example, take one **capsule** twice a day), evaluating treatment benefits and risks, and understanding insurance costs and coverage.

Who Has Limited Health Literacy Skills?

Nearly 9 out of 10 adults struggle with health literacy. Even people with high literacy skills may have low health literacy skills in certain situations. For example, someone who is stressed and sick when accessing health information may have trouble remembering, understanding, and using that information.

Why Is Health Literacy Important?

Health literacy involves more than reading—it also includes specific skills, like **calculating** the right dose of a medicine, following directions for **fasting** before surgery, or checking a nutrition label to make sure an item is safe for someone with a food **allergy**. People with low health literacy skills may have trouble doing these things.

People with low health literacy skills are more likely to have poor health outcomes, including hospital stays and emergency room visits; make medication errors; have

New Expressions	
discern /dɪ'sɜːrn/ v. 觉察出；识别；了解	**dosage** /'doʊsɪdʒ/ n. 剂量
wellness /'welnəs/ n. 健康	**capsule** /'kæpsjuːl/ n.（装药物的）胶囊
numeracy /'nuːmərəsi/ n. 数学基础知识；识数；计算能力	**calculate** /'kælkjuleɪt/ v. 计算；核算
	fast /fæst/ v. 节食；禁食；斋戒
blood sugar 血糖	**allergy** /'ælərdʒi/ n. 变态反应；过敏反应

trouble managing chronic diseases; and skip preventive services, like **flu shots**. People with higher health literacy skills are more likely to make informed health decisions. That means they are more likely to be healthy—and even to live longer.

How Can We Address Health Literacy?

Communicating clearly with people helps them find and understand health information. And when people understand health information, they can make well-informed health decisions. We can also consider taking these steps to address health literacy:

- Ensure that people in the community can easily access the health information they need.

- Create and provide plain language health materials in different languages.

- Provide training to teach health professionals and others who provide health information about health literacy **best practices**.

- Create **clearing houses** of information about health literacy for health professionals.

- Review health materials (like insurance forms and medication instructions) with community members to help make sure they understand the information—and what actions they need to take.

New Expressions		
flu shot 流感预防针	**clearing house**	信息交换机构；信息交流所
best practice 最佳做法		

Notes

1. **the U.S. Department of Health and Human Services (HHS):** 美国卫生与公众服务部。其使命是通过提供有效的卫生和社会服务，提高美国人的健康和福祉。The mission of the U.S. Department of Health and Human Services (HHS) is to enhance the health and well-being of all Americans, by providing effective health and human services and by fostering sound, sustained advances in the sciences underlying medicine, public health, and social services.

2. **Healthy People 2030:** 美国《健康公民 2030》战略规划。该规划旨在确定公共卫生优先事项，以帮助美国各地的个人、组织和社区改善健康和福祉。Healthy People 2030 is a national initiative that identifies public health priorities to help individuals, organizations, and communities across the United States improve health and well-being.

3. **the Teach-Back method:** 反馈教学法。这是一种检查患者理解情况的方法，它要求患者用自己的语言陈述保持身体健康需要了解或做的事，旨在确认患者是否理解医生所解释的健康信息。The Teach-Back method is a way of checking understanding by asking patients to state in their own words what they need to know or do about their health. It is a way to confirm that the doctors have explained things in a manner that patients can understand.

4. **the National Association of Secondary School Principals:**（美国）全国中学校长协会。这是一家非营利性组织，为初高中校长、副校长和其他学校领导提供服务。The National Association of Secondary School Principals (NASSP) is a nonprofit organization providing services to middle level and high school principals, assistant principals, and aspiring school leaders.

Post-reading Activities

I Speaking Practice: Group Discussion

Directions: *Please discuss the following questions in small groups. After your discussion, please share your opinions with the whole class.*

1. How do you understand the term "health literacy"?

2. What is digital health literacy? Why is it important for individuals living in the 21st century?

3. As medical students, what can you do to enhance health literacy in patients? Please give examples to illustrate your ideas.

II Speaking Practice: Oral Presentation

Directions: *Health literacy is an important skill based on which individuals need to manage their health. It is reported that people with higher levels of health literacy are more likely to have better health outcomes. Please search for information about health literacy levels in the Chinese population and then give an oral presentation to the whole class.*

Part 2 Thematic Reading

Health Literacy in Primary Care Practice[1]

Health literacy is the degree to which individuals have the capacity to obtain, process, and understand basic health information and services. The wide range of skills that comprise health literacy and influence a patient's ability to navigate the health care system and make appropriate decisions about his/her health include reading, writing, numeracy, communication, and, increasingly, the use of electronic technology.

More than one-third of U.S. adults, an estimated 80 million persons, have limited health literacy, making it more difficult for them to read, understand, and apply health information (e.g. wording on medication bottles, food labels, appointment slips, discharge instructions, informed consent documents, medical forms, insurance applications, medical bills, and health education materials). Although U.S. adults on average read at an eighth-grade level, more than 75% of patient education materials are written at a high school or college reading level.

Physicians often overlook health literacy in routine patient care, overestimating patients' health literacy skills and incorrectly assuming that health information and instructions have been understood. In addition, most patients fail to identify their own deficiencies in comprehension and overestimate their recall of important information.

Numerous studies with varying methodological strengths have shown that deficiencies in health literacy contribute to poor health outcomes (higher mortality rates

New Expressions	
appointment slip　预约单	**methodological** /ˌmeθədəˈlɑːdʒɪkl/ *adj.* 方法的；方法论的
routine /ruːˈtiːn/ *adj.* 常规的；例行公事的；日常的	**mortality** /mɔːrˈtæləti/ *n.* 死亡数量；死亡率

---

① The text is adapted from the following source: Hersh, L. et al. 2015. Health literacy in primary care practice. *American Family Physician*, 92(2): 118–124.

and worse overall health status), health disparities, and increased costs. The implications of health literacy are amplified in an increasingly complex and fragmented health care system that places growing demands on patients for self-care, care coordination, and system navigation. Shorter hospital stays, **polypharmacy**[1], multiple health care providers, and the rising **prevalence** of chronic disease all contribute to the increasing role that patients have in managing their own care. With this increased responsibility, limited health literacy has been associated with decreased cancer screening and immunization rates, more emergency department use, and higher rates of medication errors.

Research on health literacy interventions has shown **inconsistent** results about the extent to which they improve long-term health outcomes. However, systematic reviews of interventions designed to improve different aspects of health literacy show an overall benefit of clear health communication strategies to optimize patient care. These strategies entail improving verbal and written approaches, along with increased sensitivity to how **numerical** data are presented.

Organizations, such as **the American Medical Association**[2] and **the Agency for Healthcare Research and Quality**[3] **endorse** adopting universal health literacy **precautions** (i.e. using easy-to-understand concepts and terms with all patients instead of focusing only on those with low literacy) to minimize the risk that an individual patient will not understand the information he/she is given.

Recommendations for Enhancing Communication with Patients

Verbal Communication

Clinician-patient communication is a key component of patient care. Patients understand and **retain** about one-half of what is discussed in clinical encounters, and many do not feel comfortable asking for **clarification** or **reiteration**. With this in mind, the following strategies can be employed to promote clear and effective communication:

New Expressions	
prevalence /'prevələns/ *n.* 流行；盛行	**precaution** /prɪˈkɔːʃn/ *n.* 预防措施；预防；防备
inconsistent /ˌɪnkənˈsɪstənt/ *adj.* 不一致的；相矛盾的	**retain** /rɪˈteɪn/ *v.* 保持；继续容纳
numerical /nuːˈmerɪkl/ *adj.* 数字的；用数字表示的	**clarification** /ˌklærəfɪˈkeɪʃn/ *n.* 澄清；说明，阐明
endorse /ɪnˈdɔːrs/ *v.* （公开）赞同，支持，认可	**reiteration** /riˌɪtəˈreɪʃn/ *n.* 重述；重复

- Avoid making assumptions about language preferences or literacy levels. A patient's preferred language should be ascertained from the patient. If a clinician is unable to communicate effectively in the patient's preferred language, a trained interpreter should be used rather than relying on family members or untrained bilingual staff. Because literacy levels cannot be determined by appearances, clinicians should never assume a patient's level of understanding.

- Use plain, nonmedical language. Clinicians often use medical jargon that patients do not understand, particularly during critical moments of patient education or while developing a treatment plan. Clinicians should speak slowly and clearly and strive to mirror a patient's vocabulary. Even patients with high literacy skills may have minimal understanding of medical terms. If a medical term is used, it should be clearly explained.

- Speak slowly and break down information into small, manageable steps. Complex instructions are more challenging to understand, remember, and follow. Information or instructions should be simplified into individual steps or units and should be concrete and specific. For example, instead of telling a patient to eat a healthier diet, a physician can offer specific suggestions, such as telling the patient to eat five servings of vegetables a day and teaching about **the plate-size method**[4]. Limiting the focus of each clinical encounter to about three key messages increases comprehension of both low- and high-literacy patients.

- Confirm patient understanding. Patients rarely disclose whether they comprehend the information presented to them. One way to assure that patients have clearly understood the information is to use the Teach-Back method. This entails the patients explaining the new information in their own words, allowing the clinician to assess for comprehension. The Teach-

New Expressions	
ascertain /ˌæsər'teɪn/ v. 查明；弄清	manageable /'mænɪdʒəbl/ adj. 可操纵的；可处理的
bilingual /ˌbaɪ'lɪŋgwəl/ adj. 会说两种语言的；双语的	serving /'sɜːrvɪŋ/ n.（供一个人吃的）一份食物
minimal /'mɪnɪml/ adj. 极小的；极少的；最小的	

Back method should be framed to assess the effectiveness of the clinician's communication rather than to test the patients' learning skills. This method has been shown to increase **glycemic control** in patients with **diabetes mellitus**[5] and improve comprehension of the informed consent process.

Printed Communication

Written materials should be used to reinforce verbal communication. Verbal and written information increases patient satisfaction and knowledge compared with verbal information alone. Written materials should be at or below a fifth- to sixth-grade reading level. Written materials should be limited to key points, avoiding unnecessary details. **Visual aids**, such as pictures, drawings, or graphs, can enhance patient understanding, particularly when clinicians are communicating risks and **probabilities**.

Numerical Data

Quantitative or numerical data have a **prominent** role in health care discussions and decisions. These data include statistics about the benefits and risks of preventive behaviors, medications, and procedures, as well as disease risks and prognoses. Many physicians **presume** that the use of numbers will empower patients to make informed decisions and adopt healthier behaviors. However, many Americans have low numeracy skills, or have difficulty understanding or processing numbers. A study of patients in an **asthma** clinic found that two-thirds of all patients (not just those with limited health literacy) did not understand what 1% meant. Furthermore, the way in which numerical data are presented influences how patients understand and act on information. Although the most effective ways to communicate numerical data are unclear, several suggested approaches to improving patients' comprehension of health-related numbers include:

- Express probabilities in terms of natural frequencies rather than **percentages**.

- Provide **absolute risks**[6] rather than **relative risks**[7]; this is particularly important when risk reduction is small.

New Expressions	
glycemic control 血糖控制	**presume** /prɪ'zuːm/ v. 假设；假定
visual aid 直观教具；视觉数据	**asthma** /'æzmə/ n. 气喘；哮喘
probability /ˌprɑːbə'bɪləti/ n. 可能性；概率	**percentage** /pər'sentɪdʒ/ n. 百分率；百分比
prominent /'prɑːmɪnənt/ adj. 重要的；显眼的；显著的；突出的	

- Avoid using only positive (gain) or negative (loss) risk **framing**, and instead use both.

- Keep time **spans** at about 10 years if possible, rather than talking about lifetime risks.

Notes

1. **polypharmacy:**（治疗一种疾病时的）复方用药，混杂给药，过多给药。患者根据病情同时使用多种药物。Polypharmacy (polypragmasia) is the simultaneous use of multiple medicines by patients for their conditions. Most commonly it is defined as regularly taking five or more medicines but definitions vary in where they draw the line for the minimum number of drugs.

2. **the American Medical Association:** 美国医学会。它是世界上的三大医学会之一，创建于 1847 年，拥有 30 多万名会员，在医学领域拥有很高的地位。Founded in 1847, the American Medical Association (AMA) is the largest and only national association of the U.S. The AMA has always followed its mission: to promote the art and science of medicine and the betterment of public health.

3. **the Agency for Healthcare Research and Quality:**（美国）医疗保健研究与质量局。该机构致力于支持全美医疗有关改善质量、安全、效率和有效性的研究，通过对研究的赞助、引导和传播，帮助人们更多地知情决策并且改善医疗服务品质。The Agency for Healthcare Research and Quality's mission is to produce evidence to make health care safer, higher-quality, more accessible, equitable, and affordable, and to work within the U.S. Department of Health and Human Services and with other partners to make sure that the evidence is understood and used.

4. **the plate-size method:** 盘子法。这是一种对盘子内的食物进行划分的方法，可以让人们测量出不同食物的适当分量。The plate-size method can help people ensure their portion sizes are appropriate by keeping those higher-carb foods in smaller portions on the plate. Grains and proteins should only equal one

quarter of their plate each, while the other half should be filled with fruits and/
or vegetables.

5. **diabetes mellitus**: 糖尿病。这是一种以高血糖为特征的代谢性疾病。高血糖是由胰岛素分泌缺陷或其生物作用受损，或两者兼有引起的。Diabetes mellitus is a condition defined by persistently high levels of sugar (glucose) in the blood.

6. **absolute risks**: 绝对风险。它指某段时期发生某种疾病的可能性。Absolute risks of a disease are the risks of developing the disease over a time period. People all have absolute risks of developing various diseases, such as heart disease, cancer, stroke, etc. The same absolute risks can be expressed in different ways. For example, say you have a 1 in 10 risk of developing a certain disease in your life. This can also be said to be a 10% risk, or a 0.1 risk—depending on whether you use percentages or decimals.

7. **relative risks**: 相对风险。它指暴露组疾病发病或死亡危险与非暴露组疾病发病或死亡危险之比，亦指暴露组累积发病率或发病密度与非暴露组累积发病率或发病密度之比。Relative risk is used to compare the risk in two different groups of people. For example, the groups could be smokers and non-smokers. All sorts of groups are compared to others in medical research to see if belonging to a group increases or decreases the risk of developing certain diseases. For example, research has shown that smokers have a higher risk of developing heart disease compared to (relative to) non-smokers.

Post-reading Activities

I Language Building-up

Task 1   Extensive Vocabulary Enlargement

Directions: *The following words are taken from the text. Please follow the three-step learning in this part and build up your own Extensive Vocabulary Chart.*

Step 1. Read through the words and underline them in the text. Circle the ones that are particularly new to you. Look up the words in the dictionary and put the equivalent Chinese translation in the chart on the next page.

Step 2. While you go back to the text, please feel free to put any other words into the blanks provided in the extra lines in the chart.

Extensive Vocabulary Chart				
appointment	methodological	mortality	numerical	precaution
reiteration	bilingual	minimal	serving	glycemic
visual	probability	asthma	framing	span

Step 3. Please group the above words based on their parts of speech and meanings.

Nouns	
Verbs	
Adjectives	
Adverbs and Prepositions	
Medical Terminology	
Terminology in Other Fields	

Directions: *The following 10 words are chosen from the text. They will form the intensive vocabulary in this unit. For intensive vocabulary, you are supposed to be able to explain them in English and use them in sentence and discourse constructions.*

Step 1. Please read through the words and be familiar with their Chinese and English definitions. Recall where and how they are used in the text.

No.	Word	Translation	Definition	Status
		Intensive Vocabulary Chart		
1	routine	常规的；例行公事的；日常的	*adj.* done or happening as a normal part of a particular job, situation, or process	☆ ☆ ☆ ☆ ☆
2	prevalence	流行；盛行	*n.* the quality of existing or being very common at a particular time or in a particular place; being widespread	☆ ☆ ☆ ☆ ☆
3	inconsistent	不一致；相矛盾	*adj.* If two statements, etc. are inconsistent, or one is inconsistent with the other, they cannot both be true because they give the facts in a different way.	☆ ☆ ☆ ☆ ☆
4	endorse	（公开）赞同，支持，认可	*v.* to say publicly that you support a person, statement, or course of action	☆ ☆ ☆ ☆ ☆
5	retain	保持；继续容纳	*v.* to continue to hold or contain sth.	☆ ☆ ☆ ☆ ☆
6	clarification	澄清；说明，阐明	*n.* the act of making sth. clearer or easier to understand, or an explanation that makes sth. clearer	☆ ☆ ☆ ☆ ☆
7	ascertain	查明；弄清	*v.* to find out the true or correct information about sth.	☆ ☆ ☆ ☆ ☆
8	manageable	可操纵的；可处理的	*adj.* possible to deal with or control	☆ ☆ ☆ ☆ ☆
9	prominent	重要的；显眼的；显著的；突出的	*adj.* important; easily seen	☆ ☆ ☆ ☆ ☆
10	presume	假设；假定	*v.* to suppose that sth. is true, even without actual proof	☆ ☆ ☆ ☆ ☆

Step 2. Please tick the status for each word based on your own situation. If one word is very new or difficult for you, please tick five stars. Likewise, if one word is comparatively easy for you and you don't have to spend too much time on reading and learning it, then tick one star. The number of stars represents the difficulty of commanding the word in your eyes.

Step 3. Please complete the following 10 sentences by choosing appropriate words from the Intensive Vocabulary Chart. Please change the forms of the words where necessary.

1. The witnesses' statements were _____.
2. I _____ that he understood the rules.
3. He was surprised by the _____ of optimism about the future.
4. The church tower was a(n) _____ feature in the landscape.
5. The fault was discovered during a(n) _____ check.
6. The Prime Minister is unlikely to _____ this view.
7. She has a good memory and finds it easy to _____ facts.
8. I am seeking _____ of the regulations.
9. Tests were conducted to _____ whether pollution levels have dropped.
10. The journey is easily _____ in half an hour.

Task 3　Expressions and Sentences

Directions: *The following sentences are taken from the text. In each sentence, there is one phrase being underlined. Please refer to the dictionary and write down the explanation of the phrase in the line entitled "Meaning Exploration". After that, please make a sentence with it. Write the sentence in the line entitled "Sentence Making".*

Sentence 1

Original Sentence	The implications of health literacy are amplified in an increasingly complex and fragmented health care system that <u>places</u> growing <u>demands on</u> patients for self-care, care coordination, and system navigation.
Meaning Exploration	*place demands on:*
Sentence Making	

Sentence 2

Original Sentence	With this increased responsibility, limited health literacy has been associated with decreased cancer screening and immunization rates, more emergency department use, and higher rates of medication errors.
Meaning Exploration	*be associated with*:
Sentence Making	

Sentence 3

Original Sentence	These strategies entail improving verbal and written approaches, along with increased sensitivity to how numerical data are presented.
Meaning Exploration	*entail doing*:
Sentence Making	

Sentence 4

Original Sentence	Clinicians should speak slowly and clearly and strive to mirror a patient's vocabulary.
Meaning Exploration	*strive to*:
Sentence Making	

Sentence 5

Original Sentence	Written materials should be limited to key points, avoiding unnecessary detail.
Meaning Exploration	*be limited to*:
Sentence Making	

II Critical Reading and Thinking

Task 1 Overview and Comprehension

Directions: *The text could be divided into three small parts. Please write down the main information provided in each part based on your reading.*

Reading Notes	
Introduction	
Limited Health Literacy in Patients and Its Consequences	
Recommendations for Enhancing Communication with Patients	

Task 2 Reflection and Discussion

Directions: *After reading, please reflect on the theme of the text. Work in groups and share your opinions on the following questions with other group members.*

1. The authors pointed out that more than one-third of U.S. adults have limited health literacy. What is likely to be the situation in China based on your knowledge?

2. What are the possible consequences of limited health literacy for an individual? Please give examples to illustrate your points.

3. What strategies are recommended for doctors to promote clear and effective verbal communication with patients? Please describe the details.

4. What can doctors do to facilitate patients' understanding of numbers and statistics in primary care consultations? Please give examples to illustrate your points.

Part 3 Extended Reading

E-health Literacy in Older Adults[①]

Older adults have a higher risk of disease and decline in physical function as they age; moreover, they may experience many acute and chronic problems requiring continuous management by various medical professionals in different environments. In addition, the global **life expectancy** in 2019 was 73.4 years, and healthy life expectancy was 63.7 years. In this context, older adults likely **prioritize** a healthy life over a mere **extension** of their **lifespan**. Further, many older adults seek health information to maintain their health and treat diseases. However, although health information is provided through various channels, it is difficult for older adults to understand and manage their health using health information without proper guidelines or interventions because of its complexity. Therefore, it is essential to understand the basic literacy related to health information of older adults.

Since the 1990s, access to health information has increased due to developments in **information and communications technology (ICT)**[1]. Moreover, since then, the terms "e-health" "ehealth", and "electronic health" have appeared in literature. In the 2000s, electronic health was defined as the use of emerging ICT, especially the Internet, to improve or enable health and health care. Today, e-health has been broadly expanded to include service contents, health care providers, health consumers, and systems. Thus, the need for e-health using ICT has increased, and the role of e-health information is becoming more important.

New Expressions	
life expectancy 预期寿命	扩大）的事物
prioritize /praɪˈɔːrətaɪz/ v. 优先处理	**lifespan** /ˈlaɪfspæn/ n. 寿命
extension /ɪkˈstenʃn/ n. 延长；扩大；延长（或	

---

① The text is adapted from the following source: Jung, S. O. et al. 2022. E-health literacy in older adults: An evolutionary concept analysis. *BMC Medical Informatics and Decision Making*, *22*(1): 1–13.

 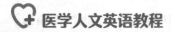

The growth in the community-**dwelling** older adult population and their expectations for patient-centered services have increased the need for the development and use of new information technologies. Older adults can now access health information using the Internet due to the wide availability of smartphones and **tablets**. While older adults started using the Internet later than younger generations, their usage is increasing rapidly with greater access to computers and the Internet. Furthermore, health information technology use among older adults in the United States of America has increased by about 19%, from 24.8% in 2009 to 43.9% in 2018. Given that the prevalence of health problems is higher in older adults than in young adults, seeking and utilizing health information over the Internet can be particularly beneficial to them. E-health information can increase access, especially for older people living in isolated rural communities. Older adults can use the Internet to help manage their health, such as making health-related decisions by searching for health information, communicating with medical professionals, seeking health services, and participating in health programs.

Early establishment of e-health mostly referred to health service and systems rather than the health of individuals. Since 2010, due to the expansion of electronic health resources to websites, web-based applications, and mobile applications, an imbalance in access to health and medical resources has occurred. Health consumers who have difficulties accessing e-health information showed a **marked** difference in appropriate self-care and self-management of their conditions. Therefore, older adults should use the Internet to identify health information to manage, maintain, and improve their own health and health care.

The term "health literacy" was first used in the United States in 1974 to refer to guidelines for health education among students. It was defined as an individual's ability to obtain, process, and understand basic health information and services necessary to make appropriate health decisions. Norman and Skinner proposed an e-health literacy model, defining e-health literacy as the ability to seek, find, understand, and appraise health information from electronic sources. According to this model, e-health literacy includes all aspects of **traditional literacy**[2] and numeracy, media, computer, information,

---

New Expressions

dwell /dwel/ v. 居住；栖身
tablet /'tæblət/ n. 平板电脑

marked /mɑːrkt/ adj. 显而易见的；明显的；显著的

and **science literacy**[3], including traditional health literacy. With the further development of information, the field of e-health has been broadly expanded from service contents, providers, users, and other major systems, and the term "digital health" has recently been widely used. According to the WHO definition, digital health encompasses emerging fields, such as big data, **genomics**, and the use of advanced computing science in **artificial intelligence** as well as **mHealth**[4] and e-health. However, e-health literacy is an important indicator of personal health technology utilization. If the level of e-health literacy is low, it is considered that it will be difficult to have digital health literacy. Therefore, rather than taking a technical approach, we would like to focus on e-health literacy at the individual level to identify the determinants of the promotion of health management for older adults and to provide a strategy to make good use of e-health resources.

We conducted a **concept analysis**[5] to confirm the meaning and attributes of e-health literacy among older adults using the evolutionary method to derive a conceptual definition of e-health literacy for older adults. The main attributes identified in this study were active information seeking, two-way interactive communication, and information utilization and sharing; moreover, we confirmed that these attributes were **organically** related. Therefore, e-health literacy of older adults can be defined as actively searching for necessary health information using electronic media, exchanging **real-time** information, and promoting one's own health by utilizing and sharing it. Therefore, based on these research results regarding e-health literacy, follow-up studies on **measurement** development and additional research are needed to reveal changes in concepts that evolve with the development of electronic resources in the future.

New Expressions

genomics /dʒə'noʊmɪks/ *n.* 基因组学

artificial intelligence 人工智能

organically /ɔːr'gænɪkli/ *adv.* 有机地；统一地；关联地

real-time /ˌriːəl 'taɪm/ *adj.* 实时的

measurement /'meʒərmənt/ *n.* 测量；度量

医学人文英语教程

1. **information and communications technology (ICT):** 信息和通信技术。它是信息技术与通信技术相融合而形成的一个新概念和新技术领域，不只局限于信息和通信技术本身，还包括消费电子产品、测量和控制仪器设备，以及电子元器件等产品、技术及其关联服务。Information and communications technology (ICT) refers to all the technology used to handle telecommunications, broadcast media, intelligent building management systems, audiovisual processing and transmission systems, and network-based control and monitoring functions.

2. **traditional literacy:** 传统读写能力。The definition of traditional literacy is the ability to read and write.

3. **science literacy:** 科学素养。国际上，人们普遍将科学素养概括为三个组成部分，即了解科学知识、了解科学的研究过程和方法、了解科学技术对社会和个人所产生的影响。Science literacy is knowledge of science, as well as the scientific framework by which people make decisions based on facts, research, and knowledge, not on opinion or hearsay.

4. **mHealth:** 移动医疗，移动健康。它是指通过移动设备提供与医疗相关的服务。MHealth is an abbreviation for mobile health, a term used for the practice of medicine and public health supported by mobile devices. The term is most commonly used in reference to using mobile communication devices, such as mobile phones, tablet computers and personal digital assistants (PDAs), and wearable devices, such as smart watches, for health services, information, and data collection.

5. **concept analysis:** 概念分析。概念分析是一种用于考察概念语义结构的方法，其目的是确定所研究概念的关键属性或特征。Concept analysis is a strategy used for examining concepts for their semantic structure. Although there are several methods for conducting concept analysis, all of the methods have the purpose of determining the defining attributes or characteristics of the concept under study.

Post-reading Activities

I   Speaking Practice: Interview

Directions: *While the Internet provides a convenient way for people to identify health information to manage, maintain, and improve their own health, older adults may still face considerable challenges in using such digital information due to their limited e-health literacy. Please work in pairs. Imagine one of you is an interviewee, a senior citizen who is new to e-health apps run on smartphones, and the other is an interviewer who interviews the senior citizen about his/her difficulties in using such apps. Please design three interview questions and take turns to be the interviewer and the interviewee.*

Interview questions:

1. _____

2. _____

3. _____

II   Reflective Writing Practice: Mini-research Project

Directions: *Based on your reading and discussion, please follow the given steps and conduct a small-scale research project on health literacy in older adults with your group members. Complete the following Research Report by filling out your major findings. Then reflect on your findings and write a short essay entitled "Health Literacy in Older Adults". The word limit is suggested to be 150–200 words.*

Research Report	
Research Objective	To investigate health literacy in older adults
Research Methods	Questionnaire and interview
Research Procedures	1. Search and read literature on health literacy in older adults. 2. Design a questionnaire in reference to the prior literature and in response to your research objective.

Research Report	
	3. Design an interview outline for deeper investigation of older adults' heath literacy. 4. Send at least 30 questionnaires and collect them. 5. Interview at least five individuals. 6. Analyze the data.
Research Findings	Please summarize the findings based on your data analysis.